# LEARN THE FACTS
# ABOUT KIDNEY DISEASE

by Steven Rosansky, MD

The information contained in this book is intended for general informational purposes only and should not be construed as medical advice from the author. This book is not intended to serve as a replacement for personal medical advice provided by your treating physician. All matters pertaining to your physical health should be supervised by your own health care providers. These professionals can provide you with the medical care that is most appropriate for your individual needs and your particular set of clinical and personal circumstances. You should never make treatment decisions on your own without consulting your physician. Any treatment decisions regarding your kidney disease should be made after joint discussions between you, your family, and your kidney treatment team. This book is recommended as a resource for these joint discussions. However, the information, research, and diet discussed in this book may not be appropriate for all patients. Therefore, a health care professional should be consulted regarding your specific situation, and the author is not liable for any medical decisions made based on the contents of this book. Any use of the information contained in this book is at the reader's discretion, and the author specifically disclaims any and all liability arising directly or indirectly from the use or application of any information contained in this book, including but not limited to any actual, special, incidental, consequential, or any other form of damages and/or liability.

*I dedicate this book to my mentor and long time friend- the late Dr. Bernie Nidus and to the wonderful patients and their families, that I have had the honor and pleasure of caring for during my 50 year career.*

# TABLE OF CONTENTS

Acknowledgments                                                        vi

Preface                                                               vii

Introduction                                                            1

**Part 1: What All Kidney Patients Should Know**                        7

  Chapter 1. The Basics of Kidney Anatomy and Function        9

  Chapter 2. How to Lower Your Risk of Atherosclerosis, Also Known as
    "Hardening of the Arteries"                      25

  Chapter 3. The Smart Diet for CKD                           39

  Chapter 4. Reversible Declines in Kidney Function           55

  Chapter 5. What You Can Do to Slow the Decline of
    Your Kidney Function                             65

Part 2: Keeping Healthy as Long as Possible Without Dialysis           85

  Chapter 6. A Look into the Crystal Ball: How Likely Is It that You
    Will Need Dialysis in the Future?                87

  Chapter 7. Electrolyte and Diuretic Management in Advanced CKD 95

  Chapter 8. Treatment of the Anemia and Bone Disease
    Associated with Advanced CKD                    111

Part 3: Preparing for Renal Replacement Therapy                       123

  Chapter 9 The Timing of Dialysis-- at a Lower eGFR
    May be the Preferred Approach                   125

  Chapter 10 Preparing for Renal Replacement Therapy:
    Kidney Transplantation, Dialysis, and Dialysis Access   139

Chapter 11 Dr. Ro's Pearls of Wisdom                                  163

Glossary                                                              185

References                                                            195

Index                                                                 221

# ACKNOWLEDGMENTS

I HAVE MANY COLLEAGUES to thank for helping me develop the clinical and research interests that led to this book. These highly acclaimed kidney specialists include Richard Glassock, UCLA; Ann O'Hare, University of Washington; Paul Eggers, NIDDK; David Goldfarb, NYU; David Harris, University of Sydney; Shang-Jyh Hwang, Kaohsiung Medical University; Brian Rayner, University of Cape Town; Robert Steiner, UCLA; Li Zuo, Peking University; Louise M. Moist, London Health Sciences Centre; Hugh Rayner, Birmingham Heartlands Hospital; Jeffrey Berns, University of Pennsylvania; Kunihiro Yamagata, University of Tsukuba; Cecile Couchoud, REIN registry; Giovanni Cancarini, University of Brescia; Manjula Kurella Tamura, Stanford University; Tanya Green, KDIGO; Kirby Jackson, USC; and Deidra Crews, Johns Hopkins.

I also want to thank my family, friends, and staff who have inspired and encouraged me to write this book, especially Alice Griffin, Arnold Bremen, Stan Dubinsky, Richard Goldstein, David Reisman, Jonathan Case, Alma Sampson, Nancy Marshall, and Brenda Rickards and my five children.

# PREFACE

I WAS MOTIVATED TO write this book on chronic kidney disease (CKD) because of three factors: The first is the campaign by kidney doctors to get everyone to know their kidney number. This number, called eGFR, is used to designate one of the five stages of CKD. In my opinion, although well intentioned, the five stages of CKD create an enormous amount of unnecessary fear. It's important to know that your kidney number can vary a lot. For example, an eGFR of 50 can be 45 or 55 on follow-up labs without any real change in your kidney function. Many CKD patients have stable kidney function for ten years or more despite these minor eGFR variations.

The second factor is that I disagree with kidney doctors who encourage the start of dialysis at progressively higher levels of a patient's own kidney function. My research, and that of many of my colleagues, shows that an earlier start of dialysis may actually be harmful. By early start, we mean starting dialysis when you have more than around 10 percent of your own kidney function remaining. Patients who start dialysis later, when they have around 5 to 10 percent or even less than 5 percent of their own kidney function, may actually survive longer than patients who start dialysis when they have higher levels of their own kidney function. My hope is that by writing this book, I can help patients avoid months, or even years, of unnecessary dialysis!

The third factor that motivated me to write this book is

the enormous amount of misinformation on CKD online and in books. Almost every book promotes a low-protein diet, and many promote the use of dietary supplements and very-low-protein diets. A low-protein diet may be right for some—but not all—kidney patients. Since kidney function remains stable for the vast majority of patients with stage 1, 2, and 3 CKD (with eGFRs above 30, see chapter 1), a low and especially a very-low-protein intake risks malnutrition, with little to no gain for many patients. Roughly half of all CKD patients are diabetic. Very-low-protein diets have not been shown to help slow decline in kidney function in diabetics. The international kidney doctor organization, Kidney Disease Improving Global Outcomes (KDIGO), referenced throughout this book does not feel that dietary protein restriction is appropriate treatment for diabetics with all stages of CKD who are not on dialysis.

# INTRODUCTION

SO, YOU WERE TOLD that you have chronic kidney disease (CKD). Let me put your kidney diagnosis in perspective. You have lots of company. One out of ten adults have CKD. Worldwide, there are 850 million patients with CKD, and 2 million patients on dialysis. In the United States, more than 130,000 patients start dialysis every year. If you are over age sixty, you have a one in four chance of having stage 3 CKD.

During my forty years as a kidney specialist, I have seen a CKD diagnosis create tremendous fear and anxiety in patients. Yet few patients truly understand what this diagnosis means and it was my duty as their nephrologist (a kidney doctor) to educate them. One of the main reasons I wrote this book is to eliminate your fears of what a CKD diagnosis means by educating you about kidney disease.

Another goal of this book is to provide you with information on the best ways to manage your kidney disease and help you separate fact from fiction. Many books and online resources that you might consider to help with your kidney problem claim that a low-protein diet can prevent your kidney function from declining and keep you off dialysis. But the fact is that randomized controlled trials, which are the gold standard for research, do not show a clear benefit of low-protein diets on preventing renal disease from progressing. The long-term follow-up of patients in the largest study, who were on a very-low-protein diet, showed no delay of progression to kidney failure; in fact, it showed an increased risk of death.

My book explains the scientifically proven methods to slow kidney function loss (chapter 5) as well as ways to predict if dialysis is likely or unlikely in your future (chapter 6). One size does not fit all CKD patients. As you will learn, patients who are at a high risk of a rapid loss of kidney function are generally younger and have high levels of urine protein. Younger age and higher urine protein are associated with a faster drop in kidney function. These patients may be advised to consider a very-low-protein diet, a lower target blood pressure, and a higher dose of certain blood pressure drugs. All CKD patients should consider my Smart Diet for CKD (chapter 3). A reduced protein intake is a part of this diet. The Smart Diet for CKD may not only help slow the decline of your kidney function, but it will also help you live longer by improving your blood pressure, decreasing obesity, decreasing your risks of the hardening of your arteries, decreasing your risk of diabetes, and decreasing your risk of colon cancer. Many books for CKD patients offer recipes, and in chapter 3 I will direct you to free kidney patient recipes.

Most patients and many clinicians are not aware of why the stages of CKD were created. One of the major reasons is for you and your physician to know that with any stage of CKD you are at a higher risk of hardening of your arteries. Progressive artery disease can shorten your life by increasing your chances of heart attack, stroke, and decreased blood flow to your legs. Good control of the risk factors that promote hardening of your arteries (see chapter 2) can help you live longer and also slow the decline of your kidney function. These lifestyle changes are much more beneficial for CKD patients than the possible benefit of low and very-low-protein diets.

For patients with CKD, herbal and other dietary supplements, promoted by some books and online sources, may be dangerous and should be avoided. Supplements are not regulated in the United States by the Food and Drug Administration (FDA), they do not have safety checks during their manufacture, and they may include impurities and other dangerous substances. For example, aristolochic acid, a Chinese herb, can cause a rapid decline in kidney function and can cause kidney cancer, yet it is still widely available in many supplements. One simple substance that most of you have in your kitchen that can be beneficial, however, is baking soda: sodium bicarbonate. Baking soda is cheap and may actually help slow the decline of kidney function as well as improve your nutrition, improve diabetes control (see chapter 7), and decrease the bone disease associated with CKD (see chapter 8).

The book is organized into three parts: The first is for patients with all stages of CKD, the second is for patients with a moderate to severe decrease in kidney function, and the third part is for patients who need to decide about dialysis or a kidney transplant. Regardless of the stage of your kidney disease, you will find information that you can use now, or later on if your kidney disease progresses.

Here is some good news: Most patients with CKD have a very mild form of the disease. Although your kidneys may not be "normal," you have plenty of kidney function left. If you have stage 1, 2, or 3 CKD, it is very unlikely that you will need dialysis in your lifetime. Even if you have one of the later stages of CKD, stage 4 or 5, fewer than one in ten patients from that group end up needing dialysis.

When I tell patients that they have kidney disease, many wonder why they don't have any symptoms and whether they did something wrong that resulted in CKD. In fact, it has been estimated that nine out of ten patients with CKD are not aware of their diagnosis. For most patients, CKD does not cause any symptoms and is just found because of a lab result (see chapter 1). It's important to know there is nothing you did "wrong" in order to cause CKD. The next thing patients wonder about is whether their kidney function can recover. More good news. In many cases, the decline in your kidney function is just temporary and is fully reversible. One of the first things to ask your kidney doctor is whether you have a reversible drop in your kidney function (see chapter 4).

For patients whose kidney disease progresses, I offer ways to stay as healthy as possible for as long as possible without dialysis. For those who face a dialysis decision, my book can help you avoid starting dialysis too soon. Many patients start dialysis early, while they still have significant amounts of their own kidney function. My research and that of my colleagues shows that a later start of dialysis may offer you the longest survival. A later start can save some patients months or even years of dialysis. If dialysis or a kidney transplant becomes necessary, I will explain the treatment options that will allow you to live the longest, with the best quality of life.

Many of you may not be prepared to read this book from cover to cover. With this in mind, "Dr Ro's Pearls of Wisdom" at the back of the book presents the highlights from each of the ten preceding chapters. After reading this, you may want to go to each chapter's introduction and summary and then to the full chapters.

Some of the topics we discuss are a little complicated. I try to make the complicated issues as clear and easy to understand as I possibly can. For quick reference, I provide a glossary of medical terms at the end of the book. This will help you speak the language of your kidney treatment team to get the best results.

The references (organized by chapter) for my book are derived from what is called "peer-reviewed publications," meaning that the science behind them is as good as it gets. I include many recommendations from KDIGO, an international organization of highly respected kidney experts.

Unfortunately, several studies show that many CKD patients are not getting the treatments and medications they need for their blood pressure and blood lipids. The accepted treatments promoted by kidney doctor organizations are often not followed. The knowledge you get from this book will not only help you get the best treatments for your CKD, but it will also help you live longer and better.

# PART 1

# WHAT ALL KIDNEY PATIENTS SHOULD KNOW

THE FIRST ORDER OF business is to understand how these fist-size organs—your kidneys—operate in your body. This lesson in kidney anatomy and function sets the stage to learn what might go wrong with your kidneys. We focus on two key lab results that connect to the stages of CKD. I discuss why I am not a fan of these stages. In my view it is the speed at which your kidney function changes that is important, not your kidney function number.

The kidney function number is called estimated glomerular filtration rate, or eGFR. It is determined by a lab value called creatinine. The blood creatinine level is just a marker for how well the kidneys are working. Avoid any of the marketed supplements that claim they can lower your blood creatinine—they have no logical place in the treatment of kidney disease and may be harmful!

Anyone with kidney disease will also want to know what this diagnosis means for them. In chapter 2, we discuss one of the main reasons to know if you have CKD. The reason is simple. With any stage of CKD, your risk of hardening and narrowing of your arteries, also called atherosclerosis, goes up. I will explain what is happening in your arteries as a result of the atherosclerosis process. You will learn how changes in your lifestyle can slow the progression of atherosclerosis and actually help you to live longer. Chapter 3 focuses on what I call the "Smart Diet" for CKD patients. The Smart Diet can help decrease progressive hardening of the arteries, slow loss of kidney function, decrease the bone disease of CKD, decrease symptoms of irritable bowel syndrome, and decrease your risk of colon cancer. Taking on this change of diet for your whole family can help prevent CKD in your children.

Many kidney books promote a low-protein diet as a way to keep you off dialysis. My Smart Diet for CKD has low protein as a component for some patients. You will learn that one size won't fit all. For some patients, low-protein diets may be harmful. Dietary supplements promoted by many books for CKD patients may be dangerous and should be avoided.

Most patients with CKD will wonder if their loss of kidney function can be reversed. Chapter 4 describes situations where decreased kidney function is reversible. A term used to describe rapid declines in kidney function is acute kidney injury, or AKI. The different types of AKI and ways to prevent and reverse these declines will be discussed.

Chapter 5 focuses on ways to slow the long-term decline of your kidney function. You will learn factors that relate to faster loss of kidney function and the scientifically proven ways to slow kidney function loss. A very-low-protein diet makes sense for patients who are at a high risk of losing kidney function rapidly—these are generally younger patients and patients with high levels of urine protein.

# Chapter 1

## The Basics of Kidney Anatomy and Function

IN ORDER TO UNDERSTAND some of the treatable and reversible causes of abnormal kidney function, it is a good idea to have a picture of kidney anatomy. From there we briefly review some of the functions of the kidneys. The kidney function test that probably got you to read this book is your estimated glomerular filtration rate, eGFR. Since much of this book relates to eGFR and urine protein, the rest of this chapter will focus on these tests.

### A Simple Anatomy Lesson

Many people have the wrong idea about where the kidneys are located. You have two fist-size kidneys located on either side of your spine, below the ribs. You can feel approximately where your kidneys are located by putting your hands on your back along your lower ribs and moving them toward your spine. In most cases, the kidneys cannot be felt when your doctor examines you.

Each kidney contains about a million tiny units called nephrons (and thus the word nephrologist, for your kidney specialist, which is the kind of doctor I am). Each nephron is made up of a glomerulus and a tubule. The main kidney artery branches into smaller arteries and eventually into the tiny blood vessels that become the glomerulus. About fifty gallons of your blood flow through your glomeruli every day. These tiny glomeruli blood vessels act as a filter to produce a liquid, or filtrate. The filtrate is the glomerular filtrate. This is where the lab test glomerular filtration rate comes from. This blood filtrate empties into a tiny tubule attached to each glomerulus. Most of what goes into these tiny tubules goes back to your bloodstream through a system of tiny blood vessels around the tubules. Some stuff is added from your bloodstream back into the tubules in order to excrete waste products. What comes out of all of the tubules is your urine.

## URINE FORMATION

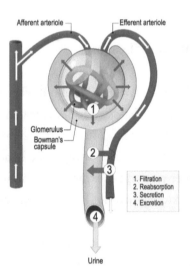

The urine from the tubules empties into a funnel-like structure (renal pelvis), which in turn connects to your ureters. Two ureters connect to your bladder. From the bladder, your urine passes out of the urethra located in the penis if you are a male and just above the vagina if you are a female. The urine system is made up of the kidneys, the ureters, the bladder, and the urethra.

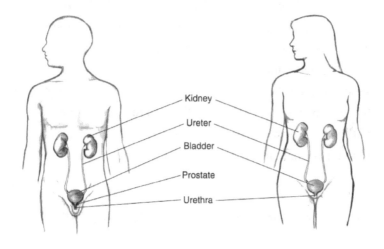

Although your kidneys get rid of waste products from your body, their most important function is to maintain the stability of the salt, water, and other components of the liquid part of your blood called the plasma.

## Some Functions of Those Remarkable Kidneys

The kidneys filter about two hundred quarts of blood a day, from which they produce one to two quarts of urine. They keep your body's fluids and salt levels in balance. The kidneys help control your blood pressure by controlling the salt and water levels in the body and by making a hormone that can narrow your blood vessels. The kidneys also make a hormone called erythropoietin, which tells the bone marrow to make more red blood cells. The kidneys make an active form of vitamin D. The kidney uses erythropoietin and a hormone called parathyroid hormone to keep your blood calcium and phosphorus levels in balance and to keep your bones strong. Finally, the kidneys help control the pH levels of the body. They can remove or add materials to your blood that can make it more or less acidic.

## Estimated Glomerular Filtration Rate—eGFR

Patients often assume that if they have CKD, they will have pain in their kidneys. This is almost never the case. For the most part, patients are not aware that they have CKD until they have a lab test that measures their urine protein or kidney function. The estimated glomerular filtration rate estimates the rate that your kidneys produce the glomerular filtrate every minute. The lab test serum creatinine is the main component of an equation that is used to get your eGFR. Small changes in serum creatinine can produce large changes in eGFR. It is important to get repeated measures of creatinine and eGFR. I have seen many patients fret over one abnormal serum creatinine or eGFR. When it's re-checked on their next visit, it is often normal. Because of the variability of your lab results, a CKD diagnosis requires the same or a lower eGFR over at least three months. A normal eGFR for young adults is around 120 to 130. For patients seventy-five or older, an eGFR of 60 may be considered normal.

*Here is an estimate of "normal" eGFR by age*

| Age | eGFR |
|---|---|
| 20–29 | 116 |
| 30–39 | 107 |
| 40–49 | 99 |
| 50–59 | 93 |
| 60–69 | 85 |
| 70+ | 75 |

## Creatinine and Home Remedies to Lower Creatinine

A fixed amount of creatinine is produced by your muscles every day. This creatinine load is excreted into your urine and provides a measure of the rate that your glomerular filtrate is produced every minute. Serum creatinine values may be lower in vegetar-ians compared to meat eaters. Older and sicker patients may be losing body muscle, the main source of creatinine, and thus can have a lower serum creatinine.

Patients may wonder what they should do about their

creatinine levels, but there is no reason to use any "natural" or home remedy to try to lower your creatinine. In fact, there is good evidence that between two patients who have the same measured kidney function, the one who has more muscle mass and a higher serum creatinine is healthier and may actually live longer!

## How to Use Serum and Urine Creatinine to Get a Measure of Kidney Function

The equations for eGFR come from research studies using creatinine data from many patients. Generally, these patients were not older, very sick, or on a low-protein or strict vegetarian diet. If you fit into any of these patient categories, your equation-derived GFR, eGFR, may be inaccurate. To get a more accurate GFR, your kidney team may need to get a measured GFR, not just an estimated GFR. One way to get a measured GFR is to get blood creatinine and a twenty-four-hour urine collection of all the creatinine that was produced over the prior day—this is a creatinine clearance. To understand creatinine clearance, you must understand how creatinine connects to glomerular filtration. The fixed amount of creatinine produced by your muscles every day is excreted into your urine. A substance that would qualify as an ideal marker of GFR cannot be removed from or added to what was filtered. The gold standard tests that give the most accurate GFR are too time consuming and expensive to be used routinely. Serum creatinine is a reasonable marker of

GFR. Very little creatinine is added to or removed from the glomerular filtrate once it is produced. By dividing the amount of creatinine in a twenty-four-hour urine collection by the serum creatinine, your doctor may be able to get a more accurate measure of your GFR, which is called your creatinine clearance.

To get your creatinine clearance, you may be asked to collect a twenty-four-hour urine sample. This twenty-four-hour urine collection is used not only to determine your creatinine clearance, but it also provides a measure of the amount of protein you spill in your urine over twenty-four hours. You can get a quick estimate of creatinine clearance if you divide your serum creatinine into one hundred. If your serum creatinine is 4 your creatinine clearance is around 25. I recommend at least two twenty-four-hour urine creatinine collections. These creatinine clearance results can be used to confirm your eGFR. If there a question about the accuracy of your eGFR and dialysis is being considered, ask to have your creatinine clearance checked at least two times.

You might ask, "So why don't we just do away with the eGFR and get creatinine clearances as the routine kidney function test?" Creatinine clearance requires an accurate twenty-four-hour collection of your urine. This is difficult for some patients, especially those who work out of the house. It is a much more expensive and more complicated way to follow your CKD, compared to following your eGFR.

## How to Collect a Twenty-Four-Hour Urine Sample

It is much easier to get these spot urine tests than it is to get a twenty-four-hour urine. If done correctly, a twenty-four-hour urine can be helpful to get a measured kidney function and total daily protein excretion. To get an accurate twenty-four-hour urine, start the collection in the morning after you go to the bathroom. Collect all your urine the rest of the day. Be sure to include the next morning's urine sample when you get up. Then you are done.

## Protein in the Urine

The second key measure of your kidney's health is protein in your urine. The speed with which your kidney function declines is best predicted by the level of protein in your urine. Protein in the urine is also called proteinuria. Normal glomeruli allow very little protein to pass through. Kidney diseases can change your glomeruli and they can become "leaky" to protein that is filtered from the bloodstream.

A urinalysis consists of a urine dipstick and a look at the urine under the microscope. A quick and inexpensive way to check for protein or blood in the urine is to use the urine dipstick. This strip changes color when you have protein or blood in the urine. If you have a 1+ or less protein on the urine dipstick, you have a mild increase in urine protein. If you have a 2+ or more protein on the dipstick, this corresponds to heavier proteinuria.

An area of confusion are the terms "proteinuria" and

"albuminuria." Proteinuria is all the types of proteins that are in the urine. But albuminuria is a measure of the protein called albumin that is in the urine. Urine dipsticks are measuring the albumin, not total urine protein. The main protein in urine is albumin.

A dipstick of the urine is a good screen for albuminuria, but it is not very specific. You may be asked to give a tiny sample of your urine, also called a spot urine, to test for albumin and creatinine. The albumin to creatinine ratio, albumin/creatinine, closely estimates your twenty-four-hour urine albumin excretion. If this test result is under 30, you have normal or mildly increased urine protein; if the result is between 30 and 300 you have what is called microalbuminuria, or moderately increased urine protein. If the ratio is over 300, it is called macroalbuminuria, or severely increased urine protein. Like eGFR, it is wise to repeat this urine test a few times. The average of the results provides you with your baseline proteinuria level. These levels should be monitored a few times a year. A decline in the amount of urine protein may correlate with an improvement in the rate of kidney function loss. This is especially true if you have macroalbuminuria. Follow-up spot urine checks will help your doctor determine if your proteinuria is increasing or decreasing.

## Blood in the Urine

The urine dipstick can also check for red and white blood cells in the urine. White blood cells can indicate infection. Red blood cells may be part of disease of the glomeruli, if you also have protein in the urine. Often blood in the urine is part of diseases that the kidney surgeon—the urologist—deals with, including kidney stones and tumors of the kidneys, ureters, and bladder.

## The Five Stages of CKD (and Why I Am Not a Fan of Defining These Stages)

Stage 1 is an eGFR above 90, with an abnormal urinalysis—blood or protein in the urine.

Stage 2 is called a mild decrease in kidney function, with an eGFR of 60–89.

Stage 3 is called a moderate decrease in kidney function, with an eGFR of 30–59.

Stage 4 is called a severe decrease in kidney function, with an eGFR of 15–29.

Stage 5 is called kidney failure, with an eGFR <15. Patients who are on dialysis are also called stage 5 CKD.

The United States started a campaign to get laboratories across the world to report your eGFR. The stages of CKD were an outgrowth of this move to report eGFR. The routine reporting of eGFRs, in my opinion and that of many other kidney specialists, has created a good deal of unnecessary worry. Why do I say this? Before we had the routine reporting of eGFR, doctors relied on the serum creatinine test. As I pointed out, if you were an informed doctor, you could get a quick GFR estimate by dividing creatinine into 100. For example, if you had a serum creatinine of 1.5 that would be 100/1.5, or GFR around 66. Most doctors were not concerned with this result before we had the CKD stages. A patient with creatinine of 1.5 was not necessarily labeled as having CKD. Some doctors make the argument that we were underdiagnosing CKD. But I think the routine reporting of eGFR moved us to the other extreme of overdiagnosis and overtreatment of kidney disease.

Why do I say overdiagnosis? First, it is hard to know what is truly a normal versus a mild or moderate decrease in kidney function. For example, half of all patients over seventy-five have a moderate decrease in eGFR (stage 3 CKD, eGFR 30–60). In my opinion, and in the opinion of many of my colleagues, if you are over seventy-five with an eGFR of 30–60, your eGFR may be compatible with your age and may not mean that you have CKD. Also, the accuracy of an eGFR level that is above 60 is relatively poor. To me if you have an eGFR above 60, with no protein or blood in your urine, you do not have a serious CKD problem.

If you search the web for the CKD stages, you will find some crazy stuff. One site says, "if you have stage 4 CKD, you may feel quite ill and get jaundice." Neither of these statements is correct. Kidney disease is not associated with jaundice, and most patients with stage 4 CKD do not have significant symptoms.

One of my biggest problem with stages of CKD relates to the issue of when to start dialysis. Many web searches will tell you that stage 5 CKD (eGFR below 15) is end-stage renal disease. You may also be told in your search that if you have stage 5 CKD, you need a kidney transplant or dialysis. I disagree with both of these statements.

In chapter 9, I discuss the trend to start patients on dialysis at progressively higher eGFRs. One of the factors that contributed to earlier start of dialysis (at higher eGFRs) is the notion that an eGFR of less than 15 represents renal failure, also sometimes referred to as end-stage renal failure. To me a patient is "end stage" when they have a level of eGFR where they truly need dialysis or a kidney transplant. The need for dialysis and being "end stage" should be based on clinical symptoms, not just an eGFR level. For most patients this occurs at an eGFR of less than 10, and for some patients at an eGFR of less than 5.

### The Latest CKD Staging Includes Urine Protein

As we will discuss in greater detail, both your eGFR level and your urine protein level can independently increase your risk of hardening of your arteries (atherosclerosis) and progressive CKD. With this in mind, the latest kidney disease classification includes both your eGFR and urine protein level (albuminuria). The staging also splits CKD 3 into two groups.

*The Six Categories of eGFR Under the New System Are:*
G1: same as CKD stage 1, eGFR over 90, considered normal
G2: same as CKD stage 2, eGFR 60–89, mildly decreased kidney
  function
G3a: mild to moderately decreased kidney function at eGFR 45–59
G3b: moderately to severely decreased kidney function at eGFR
  30–44
G4: same as CKD 4, severely decreased kidney function at eGFR
  15–29

G5: same as CKD 5, kidney failure, eGFR less than 15

This staging also classifies three levels of spot urine protein (albuminuria):

A1: normal to mildly increased, less than 30

A2: moderately increased, 30–299

A3: severely increased, 300 or more

This new CKD staging is a little better than the old classifications since it places an emphasis on both eGFR as well as urine protein. The urine protein levels are scored by A1 to A3 categories. So in the new staging, you have a G stage for your eGFR and an A stage for the urine protein. It turns out that even if you have a normal eGFR, if your urine protein level is severely increased (A3), you may develop more severe atherosclerosis and CKD complications than a patient with an eGFR of 30–60 without proteinuria. Unfortunately, the new classification scheme continues to call CKD 5, now called G5, kidney failure. By using this term, many patients and clinicians might assume that once eGFR reaches 15, dialysis is required. This is not the case. Splitting stage 3 into G3a (eGFR 45–59) and G3b (eGFR 30–44) makes sense if a patient has a greater risk for atherosclerosis complications and renal disease progression with CKD 3b versa 3a. Unfortunately, we do not have proof of this view.

*Note: In order to simplify our discussion, I will continue to use the old method of five stages of CKD throughout this book.*

## Frequency of CKD Stages and Recommendations for Treatment

Many of you were told that you have CKD. Those patients with early-stage CKD have much less to worry about than do patients with later-stage CKD 4 and CKD 5. As you can see from the old and new stages of CKD, stage 1 in the newer classification is normal (it's now called G1) unless a patient has a urine protein over 30. Early stages of CKD are much more common than later stages of CKD. For example, stage 1 CKD is roughly twice as common as stage 2 CKD, and stage 2 CKD is over five times more frequent than stage 3 CKD. Stage 3 CKD is about thirteen times more frequent than combined CKD stage 4 and stage 5 CKD. Thus, the vast majority of patients with CKD have CKD stage 1, 2, and 3. Patients with stage 4 and 5 CKD are twice as likely to have proteinuria category A2 and A3 (over 30) compared to patients with earlier stage CKD.

As we will discuss in chapters 3 and 5, the promotion of very-low-protein diets and diet supplements, or the aggressive use of certain medications (ACE and ARB drugs, see chapter 4) for the very large population of CKD patients with eGFRs above 30 could expose these patients to treatments that may not have any benefit and may be harmful.

## Kidney Disease Stages Versus Pattern of GFR Change

I believe that it is the pattern of your kidney function change over time that really matters. To be diagnosed hypertensive, you need repeated high blood pressure levels over the course of weeks to months. To be sure you have CKD, the decreased eGFR level must be present for at least three months. The repeated eGFR measures over months or even years are what you should be following, not any one test. Some of these eGFR results will be outliers. You should not be concerned about these outlier results. Any decision regarding your CKD management should be based on the repeated results and the pattern and speed of your eGFR change.

Some patients can have stable stage 3, 4, and even stage 5 CKD for years. Remember, even if you have stage 4 CKD, only one in ten of you may need to worry about dialysis.

If you want to get an idea of whether you will need dialysis, I refer you to chapter 6.

### SUMMARY

Your kidneys have many important functions. For the purposes of this book, the two most important aspects of kidney function are the estimated glomerular filtration rate, eGFR, and how much protein is in your urine. It is important to remember that eGFR is just a calculated estimate of your actual kidney function. To get a measure of your actual kidney function, a twenty-four-hour urine for creatinine clearance should be considered. Although not perfect, eGFR is a good estimate of kidney function. Following your eGFR is a reasonable way to follow your CKD. Levels of eGFR above 60 are less reliable than eGFR levels below 60. Levels above 60 rarely mean that you will have problems from CKD. On the other hand, even with an eGFR in the normal range, a significant amount of protein in your urine is a reason to follow your CKD more closely. Blood in the urine may also be of significance, but it is not a key component of CKD staging.

The kidneys have many other important functions. These functions will be reviewed in part 2, when we discuss the problems that may occur as kidney disease progresses. Remember, just because you have an eGFR of less than 30 (CKD 4) or even CKD 5 does not mean that you will need dialysis in the near future.

# Chapter 2

---

## How to Lower Your Risk of Atherosclerosis, Also Known as "Hardening of the Arteries"

ONE OF THE MAIN reasons to know that you have CKD is that you have an increased risk of an accelerated hardening of your arteries, also called atherosclerosis. This important fact was behind the campaign to have doctors and their patients recognize abnormal kidney function. If you take on the lifestyle changes in this chapter, there is strong evidence that you can add years to your life. And if you are a good role model for your kids in this healthy lifestyle, they too will live longer.

The most important contributors that lead to hardening of your arteries are smoking, high blood pressure, elevated blood sugar, obesity, high cholesterol, low levels of physical activity, and stress. We'll discuss each of these stressors to your arteries in this chapter, but first, let's learn more about why hardening of the arteries is so dangerous.

### What Is Atherosclerosis?

Atherosclerosis is the narrowing and hardening of your arteries from a waxy substance called plaque. Plaque and fats build up in your arteries over many years. It's a silent process and does not cause symptoms until the condition is in an advanced state. Plaque in the arteries that supply the heart—the coronary arteries—can lead to chest pain, heart attack, heart failure, arrhythmias, or even death. Plaque can build up in arteries that supply the brain, which can lead to strokes. Plaque can also accumulate in arteries to your legs. This can lead to surgical amputations.

So it's important to be aware of the warning signs: with decreased blood flow to the arteries of the heart, you may experience chest pain with increased activity. This is an important signal that you may be at risk for a heart attack. A stroke may be preceded by a change in your ability to move a part of your body—an arm or a leg—or even loss of the ability to smile, speak, or see. These symptoms may be short lived. They may be a signal of a stroke to come. With decreased blood flow to your legs, you may experience painful cramping of leg muscles while walking.

It is important for you to be aware of these warning signals. With the appropriate interventions by your medical providers, you may be able to save yourself from having a heart attack or a stroke or requiring an amputation.

## How to Reduce Your Risk of Atherosclerosis

There are many clinical and life style issues that relate to your risk of hardening of the arteries. This sections reviews these factors and suggests ways to reduce your atherosclerosis risk.

### Reduce the Protein in Your Urine

In addition to your level of eGFR, the amount of protein in your urine is a strong predictor of bad outcomes from hardening of your arteries. The most recent staging of CKD uses both your eGFR level as well as the amount of protein in your urine. Even low levels of protein in your urine (trace or 1+ on urinalysis) can place you at an increased risk of the atherosclerosis complications.

There are certain medicines that can decrease the protein in your urine. If you take these medicines as prescribed and get a decrease in your urine protein, there can be multiple benefits. One is a potential decrease in atherosclerosis complications. A second important benefit is a slowing of the decline in your kidney function. The use of these important medicines will be discussed at length in chapters 4 and 5.

### Quit Smoking

If you are currently a smoker and have CKD, I encourage you to quit smoking. Why is this so important? Smoking is the number one cause of preventable disease and death. There is no safe amount of smoking. The longer you smoke, the greater your risk. If you smoke a pack of cigarettes a day, your risk of heart attack is doubled compared to someone who does not smoke.

The good news is that if you stop smoking, you not only decrease your risk of progressive atherosclerosis, coronary heart disease, stroke, and lung cancer, but you may also slow the decline in your kidney function. You will likely add years to your life. There is a long list of other benefits soon after you quit. Your lungs function better, you have less coughing and shortness of breath, you have more energy, you are actually less stressed, fertility and sex drive improve, your senses of smell and taste get a boost, your skin looks younger, your teeth whiter, your breath sweeter, and if you have a smoke-free home, you protect your loved ones from the harms of secondhand smoke. Secondhand smoke increases risks of lung cancer, heart disease, stroke, and asthma.

There are several over-the-counter aids that may help you to decrease or eliminate cigarettes. Many patients substitute nicotine patches, nicotine gum, or nicotine lozenges for their cigarettes. There are also prescription medications your physician can prescribe to help you stop smoking. Although their use is controversial, e-cigarettes and vaping are probably less harmful than smoking. These cigarette substitutes may be beneficial as long as the e-cigarette does not contain potential harmful flavors and other substances.

There are many free programs and resources that can help you stop smoking. These resources are available from your local chapter of the American Cancer Society, American Heart Association, or the American Lung Association. You can also use online resources to help you quit smoking through many organizations, such as the Centers for Disease Control, the National Cancer Institute, the National Clearinghouse for Alcohol and Drug Information, and the World Health Organization Tobacco Free Initiative.

## Get Regular Physical Activity

Exercising at least four or five times a week decreases your risk of atherosclerosis complications. It also can improve your breathing capacity and lower your blood pressure and your cholesterol. Exercise can also help you lose weight. It is good for both your physical and emotional health, and it is a great stress reliever.

Here are some tips: Decrease your sitting time by thirty minutes every day. Shoot for decreased time in front of your TV, computer, or iPad screen. Replace this screen time with an exercise you like. Walking is a great choice. Try walking at a brisk pace. You can walk anywhere—at home, around the neighborhood, on the golf course, at the shopping mall. Some folks like to use a Fitbit to track their steps; ten thousand steps a day is a reasonable goal. Try to find an exercise partner to chat with. If walking is a problem for you because of an injury, consider a stationary bike.

Swimming is also great for those with problems walking. Many public pools offer water aerobics classes. Start your exercise slowly, fifteen minutes a day, and gradually increase your exercise to thirty minutes of moderate-intensity exercise five times a week. Any amount of physical activity will have health benefits. The more you exercise, the greater the benefits. Muscle-strengthening exercises that involve all muscle group can help counter the loss of muscle that comes with progressive CKD. If you are an older adult, try to be as physically active as you can.

## Control Your Blood Pressure

Eight out of ten patients with CKD have elevated blood pressure, so it is likely that yours is elevated as well. Most of you are familiar with blood pressure measurements taken in your doctor's office. You may also know that the normal top number, your systolic blood pressure, is around 120. The normal bottom number, diastolic blood pressure, is 80.

As a first step to managing your high blood pressure, it is important to get a picture of your blood pressure readings outside of the doctor's office or clinic. A good investment for anyone with CKD is a digital blood pressure machine. These machines are inexpensive, easy to use, and can be purchased at your local pharmacy. Try to get some readings of your blood pressure at home, at work, and before each dose of your blood pressure medicines. Give this data to your kidney treatment team. These real-life blood pressure readings will help you get proper blood pressure treatment.

You may be one of the many patients who have much higher blood pressures when you are in your doctor's office than when you are at home or at work. This is termed "white coat" hypertension. Without blood pressure readings outside of their office, your medical provider will not be aware that you have "white coat" hypertension. This can lead them to prescribe too much blood pressure medicine. Overtreatment of your blood pressure can be dangerous, as we will discuss.

Accurate blood pressure readings also depend on proper technique. You may get falsely high readings if you or your medical provider take your blood pressure after you have been very active or when you are worried. Here are some tips to get accurate blood pressures: First, relax for about five minutes. Keep your arm with the blood pressure cuff at the level of your heart. You can do this by resting your arm on a chair's arm or on a table. If your arm is large and the blood pressure cuff can't wrap around one and a quarter to one and a half times, you may need a larger blood pressure cuff. Too small a cuff can give falsely high readings.

### Achieving Your Goal Blood Pressure

The next issue to address is your goal blood pressure. It was thought in the past that the lower your blood pressure, the better. This turns out not to be true. In chapters 4 and 5, we will discuss the target blood pressures for different patients' situations. The reason that a low target blood pressure (110–20 top number) is not the goal for everyone is the possibility that too low a blood pressure can decrease the blood flow to the kidney. For some patients too low a blood pressure may accelerate the loss of kidney function. If blood pressure gets below the 90–100 systolic range, it may not only harm your kidneys, but it may also damage your heart and your brain. Low blood pressures can lead to chest pain, heart attacks, and strokes. I have been on blood pressure medication, as have many of my friends. Many of us inadvertently continued our blood pressure medication with systolic blood pressures of less than 100. I have seen how too much blood pressure medicine causes low blood pressures in my clinic, in hospitalized patients, and in my friends. This overtreatment caused patients to pass out, fall, and even led to acute kidney failure.

The best way to keep this from happening is to check your blood pressure regularly. Be sure to check your blood pressure before you take your blood pressure pills. This is especially important if you are feeling weak, light-headed, or if you are sick and can't drink enough. If your blood pressure is less than 110 systolic, you may want to hold the next dose of your blood pressure meds. You can resume taking your blood pressure meds once your systolic blood pressure is above 130. It is important for you to discuss this approach with your primary care provider.

## Do Things That Help You Relax

Try things that will reduce the stress in your life. Less stress can help you live longer, it can decrease your blood pressure, and it can lessen your risks from hardening of the arteries. Exercise is a great stress reliever. Some of my patients find that meditation can help lower blood pressure and is good for their overall health and mood. Yoga or tai chi are two forms of exercise that combine relaxation with purposeful relaxed movements.

Another factor in stress relief is to increase your social contacts. Several research studies have shown a strong correlation between social interaction and health and well-being. Social isolation may have significant adverse effects, especially for older adults.

## Get Enough Sleep

Another issue that relates to stress levels, blood pressure, and atherosclerosis is your sleep. Try to get at least eight hours of sleep every night. If you are told by a sleep partner that you have periods when you stop breathing, together with loud snoring, you may have sleep apnea. If you provide this history to your doctor, they may order a sleep study to diagnose sleep apnea. Sleep apnea increases your risk of atherosclerosis. It can make your blood pressure difficult to control. Patients with this condition may complain of feeling tired and not well rested even after eight hours of sleep. It can cause you to fall asleep very easily during the daytime. Weight loss can decrease the severity of sleep apnea.

## Lower Your Lipids, Especially Your Bad Cholesterol

Cholesterol levels have been linked to atherosclerosis. Cholesterol has two main types: "bad" cholesterol, LDL, and "good" cholesterol, HDL. Despite its name, research has shown that raising your HDL does not lower your risk of atherosclerosis-related problems. On the other hand, lowering your LDL can help decrease the plaque buildup in the walls of your arteries and prevent further blockage of these blood vessels.

All CKD patients are at an increased risk of atherosclerosis and thus should have an LDL goal of less than 100. Some clinicians aim for an LDL of less than 70, especially for diabetics with CKD. Statins are a type of medicine that can help you reach these LDL levels. Some commonly prescribed statins include Lipitor (atorvastatin), Zocor (simvastatin).

## Muscle Toxicity from Lipid Drugs with CKD

If you develop pains in your muscles after starting statins or so-called fibric acid drugs, such as Lopid (gemfibrozil) or TriCor (fenofibrate), you must stop these medicines and let your doctor know. These drugs can cause muscle breakdown in patients with decreased kidney function. These muscle-breakdown products can lead to kidney failure. For most patients, studies have shown that mild muscle or joint pains are probably not coming from the lipid-lowering drugs.

### Lose Weight

One of the factors that can increase your risk of atherosclerosis is obesity. Obese patients are more likely to become diabetic and hypertensive. There is some evidence that being overweight by itself can worsen kidney function. Many patients struggle with their weight. Here are a few weight-loss tips. The only way to achieve weight loss is to take in fewer calories than your body burns. Fewer calories in and more exercise is the formula for success. Portion sizes in most of the developed world are far too large. Simply cutting down on your portion sizes and leaving the table before you go for seconds or thirds will help. If you follow the Smart Diet for CKD (see chapter 3), you will lose weight.

**Control Your Blood Sugar**

Despite many years of study, it is still unclear whether elevated blood sugars, by themselves, increase your atherosclerosis risk. What is known regarding your blood sugar is that poor glucose control in a diabetic will increase your risk of getting the eye problems of diabetes: diabetic retinopathy. Diabetic retinopathy can lead to blindness. Poor sugar control in a diabetic who does not have CKD can increase the likelihood that you will develop CKD.

The other side of the blood sugar issue are the harms from having low blood sugars. Experts in diabetes treatment have come to realize that there is a potential for harm from too much diabetes medicine. The treatment targets for diabetics revolve around A1C levels. A1C reflects average blood sugars over approximately the past three months.

There is pretty good evidence that if you have type 1 or type 2 diabetes, an A1C of less than 7 can help to prevent an increase in urine protein and a decrease in eGFR (preventing diabetic CKD). Unfortunately, once you have diabetic CKD, lower blood sugar levels may not slow loss of eGFR.

The A1C target that will give CKD patients the best outcomes has not been established. For most patients who already have an eGFR of less than 60, a target A1C of 7 can help you avoid dangerously low blood sugars. Patients who have had a stroke or heart attack and older patients with a limited life expectancy can shoot for an A1C in the 8 range.

The reason to be concerned about low blood sugars is that in some cases patients may not be aware that their blood sugar is dropping. Usual symptoms from low blood sugar include sweating, dizziness, and trouble thinking clearly. If blood sugar gets very low for an extended period, it can cause you to pass out, have a seizure, or go into a coma. Always have hard candy or crackers available in case your blood sugar drops.

## Other Important Issues for Diabetics with CKD

Diabetes by itself increases your risk of atherosclerosis complications. Diabetes and CKD, especially CKD with high levels of urine protein, puts patients at the highest risk of getting atherosclerosis complications. Following the recommendations in this chapter can help you decrease these risks.

In addition to the lifestyle changes to reduce atherosclerosis, diabetics need to have proper foot care, which includes regular visits to the foot doctor—a podiatrist. Foot care includes daily washing and inspection of your feet. At any sign of a problem, let the podiatrist treat you. Do not try to remove calluses or other foot lesions yourself. Proper foot care can prevent the foot ulcers that often lead to amputations.

Yearly eye exams by an optometrist or ophthalmologist for early detection and treatment of diabetic eye issues can almost entirely eliminate the risk of blindness in diabetics with CKD. Vision loss can come from diabetic retinopathy (blood vessel disease in the back of the eye), glaucoma, and cataracts.

## SUMMARY

Decreased eGFR and increased urine protein individually and together increase your risk of atherosclerosis complications. This increased risk is one of the main reasons to be aware that you have a decreased eGFR and protein in your urine. To lower your risk, try to take on the lifestyle changes discussed in this chapter. I understand that making these changes requires a lot of effort. Take on as many as you can. Try to quit smoking. The benefits from this are huge and immediate. Try to get daily exercise, adequate sleep, and relaxation time. Follow a diet high in fruits, vegetables, and fiber and low in saturated fats and sugars (see chapter 3). Have your doctor monitor your bad cholesterol, your LDL. Try to reach an LDL level below 100. Diabetics with an eGFR below 60 may want to shoot for an A1C in the 7 range and an LDL below 70. Control of the atherosclerosis risk factors is even more important if you have diabetes and CKD. Keep a record of your blood pressure for yourself and your kidney treatment team. Remember that too low a blood pressure can result in a decline in your kidney function. This issue and other situations that can lead to a reversible decline in your eGFR will be reviewed in chapter 4. Chapters 4 and 5 will also explain how to decrease the protein in your urine. A decrease in your urine protein can have the combined benefit of slowing progression of atherosclerosis and slowing loss of your kidney function.

# Chapter 3

## The Smart Diet for CKD

AS WE DISCUSSED IN chapter 1, most CKD patients have an eGFR above 30 with relatively low levels of urine protein. These patients are not at a high risk for a rapid loss of kidney function. The emphasis on low-protein diets in many books on CKD for patients is, in my opinion, misguided. To me, if you have stage 1, 2, or 3 CKD, the lifestyle changes to decrease your risk of atherosclerosis (discussed in chapter 2) are much more important than a low-protein diet. My Smart Diet for CKD is "Smart" because it can help to decrease your risk of progressive atherosclerosis, slow loss of eGFR, help decrease the bone disease of CKD, decrease irritable bowel symptoms, decrease colon cancer risk, and help with control of diabetes and hypertension. It is also a "Smart" diet since it does not place extreme restrictions on any diet components—it's a diet you can actually follow. If you take on this Smart Diet for your whole family, there is a good chance that you can decrease the likelihood that other family members will get CKD.

First, we'll review how to read food labels and how to apply this to weight loss and the various components of your diet. We'll explore how each diet component may affect your kidneys and your overall health. Finally, you'll learn how the Smart Diet for CKD needs to be modified in some patients with advanced CKD and for some older patients.

## The Smart Diet

Why do I call the diet I recommend the Smart Diet for CKD? The reason is simple. As we discussed in chapter 2, a concern for everyone with any stage of CKD is progressive atherosclerosis. If you follow the Smart Diet for CKD, you can decrease your risk of atherosclerosis. The second target of the Smart Diet for CKD is its effect on the rate of loss of your kidney function. The relationship between dietary protein and loss of kidney function is discussed in chapter 5. The Smart Diet does not require a very-low-protein intake or expensive supplements that may be necessary for patients on a very-low-protein diet. In my opinion, the risk of malnutrition and the high cost of these very-low-protein diets makes my Smart Diet for CKD a much better alternative since it is relatively low in protein. The Smart Diet for CKD is high in fruits, vegetables, fiber, and fish and low in red meat. If you choose this diet, most of you will reduce your daily protein intake. My Smart Diet does not insist on a specific low-protein diet goal. On the other hand, since reducing your protein intake may slow the loss of your kidney function, the relatively low-protein intake of the Smart Diet is worth your effort. The Smart Diet for CKD will decrease your total calorie intake to help manage obesity. The Smart Diet for CKD will benefit your overall health with its reduced intake of foods with added sugar and high levels of carbohydrates, the emphasis on eating more whole grains and fewer refined grains, eating more fiber and fewer saturated fats, reducing sodium (salt) and decreasing phosphorus intake. The health benefits of each of these components of the Smart Diet for CKD are discussed below. This diet may not be appropriate for patients with advanced CKD who need to severely restrict potassium and phosphorus in their diet. If you are in this category, you will need to have a licensed dietician provide your special diet.

## Food Labels and the Smart Diet for CKD Patients

In order to eat more of the recommended foods in the Smart Diet and fewer of the foods to avoid, it helps to get used to looking at food labels.

Food labels show both a single serving (A) and what is in the whole container (B). The serving size on the label is based on the amount of food that people typically eat at one time. It also assumes a two-thousand-calorie diet, which would go along with this portion size.

When converting grams of protein, fat, or sugars to calories, use the following: A gram of protein has four calories, a gram of carbohydrates has four calories, and a gram of fat has nine calories.

The total number of calories a person needs each day varies depending on your age, sex, height, weight, and level of physical activity. In addition, a need to lose, maintain, or gain weight and other factors affect how many calories should be consumed.

A

## Nutrition Facts

8 servings per container
**Serving size** **2/3 cup (55g)**

Amount per serving
**Calories** **230**

| | % Daily Value* |
|---|---|
| **Total Fat** 8g | **10%** |
| Saturated Fat 1g | **5%** |
| Trans Fat 0g | |
| **Cholesterol** 0mg | **0%** |
| **Sodium** 160g | **7%** |
| **Total Carbohydrate** 37g | **13%** |
| Dietary Fiber 4g | **14%** |
| Total Sugars 12g | |
| Includes 10g Added Sugars | **20%** |
| **Protein** 3g | |
| Vitamin D 2mcg | 10% |
| Calcium 260mg | 20% |
| Iron 8mg | 45% |
| Potassium 240mg | 6% |

*The % Daily Value (DV) tells you how much a nutrient in
a serving of food contributes to a daily diet. 2,000 calories
a day is used for general nutrition advice.

B

## Nutrition Facts

2 servings per container
**Serving size** **1 cup (255g)**

| Calories | Per serving 220 | Per container 440 |
|---|---|---|
| | % DV* | % DV* |
| **Total Fat** | 5g  **6%** | 10g  **13%** |
| Saturated Fat | 2g  **10%** | 4g  **20%** |
| Trans Fat | 0g | 0g |
| **Cholesterol** | 15mg  **5%** | 30mg  **10%** |
| **Sodium** | 240mg  **10%** | 480mg  **21%** |
| **Total Carb.** | 35g  **13%** | 70g  **25%** |
| Dietary Fiber | 6g  **21%** | 12g  **43%** |
| Total Sugars | 7g | 14g |
| Incl. Added Sugars | 4g  **8%** | 8g  **16%** |
| **Protein** | 9g | 18g |
| Vitamin D | 5mcg  25% | 10mcg  50% |
| Calcium | 200mg  15% | 400mg  30% |
| Iron | 1mg  6% | 2mg  10% |
| Potassium | 470mg  10% | 940mg  20% |

* The % Daily Value (DV) tells you how much a nutrient in a serving of
food contributes to a daily diet. 2,000 calories a day is used for general
nutrition advice.

To get a good idea of the total daily calories you want to shoot for to maintain your weight or to lose weight slowly or quickly, go to www.healthline.com. You will need to put in your sex, age, height, and weight to get the recommended level of daily calories. It will give you the recommended calories for your age, level of activity, and whether you want to decrease your weight, increase your weight, or keep it stable. Patients who do little activity will have lower recommended daily calories. With increasing age, metabolism slows, so recommended daily calories also go down.

A decrease in portion size is essential if you want to lose weight. If you can decrease your portion size to the size recommended on the food label for a single serving, you will be on your way to losing weight. The reason I say this is that the average American eats 3,800 calories—almost twice what these labels are assuming! The United States ranks number one in the world for average daily calorie intake. The percent of daily value of the food that you read on the food labels assumes a two-thousand-calorie diet. These percent of daily values may not have a lot meaning for you, especially if you eat four thousand calories versus the assumed two thousand calories a day. My advice is to focus less on daily requirements and pay more attention to the total calories, carbohydrates, sugars, fiber, fat, cholesterol, sodium, protein, and phosphorus that you eat. Let's look at these individually.

Food labels will provide you with information on the calories, the carbohydrates, and the added sugar in your food. If you are overweight, shoot for the total daily calorie goal that you can get from www.healthline.com. Try to avoid foods with added sugars. Carbohydrates are the main source of extra calories. To lose weight, read labels to help reduce your carbohydrate intake. Food items to reduce or avoid are sweeteners like sugar, honey, and syrup and foods with added sugars like candy, cakes, ice cream, pastries, and sweetened beverages, especially sodas. Calories from sugary drinks are the most fattening aspect of the modern diet. Your brain does not register liquid calories the same way it does solid calories. For example, when you drink sugary soda, your brain will not compensate by having you eat less of other things. There is no real need for any of these sugary beverages, and their long-term harms are enormous.

By cutting carbs, you reduce your appetite and increase your speed of weight loss. A low-carb diet can also help prevent type 2 diabetes. Eating fiber-rich carbs of the Smart Diet for CKD will be your best bet. A glass of red wine daily may have health benefits. If you drink more alcohol than this, consider cutting out beer, wine, and mixed drinks, which are all very high in calories.

## Drinking Water and Weight Loss

If you do not have a need to restrict water due to advanced CKD or heart disease, a simple trick to help with weight loss is to drink more water. Try to drink the water before meals to reduce hunger and decrease your caloric intake. Caffeinated beverages like green tea and coffee are good since they may also boost metabolism.

## Diet Protein and Weight Loss

A diet that has fewer carbs and more protein has several benefits. Protein calories are more filling than carb calories. Therefore, this type of diet can reduce your appetite and cut cravings. Eating more protein and fewer carbs can also increase the calories you burn.

## Exercise and Weight Loss

If you are able to decrease your calorie intake, your body will adjust by burning fewer calories. But as you lose weight, you may lose body muscle. Your body muscle burns a lot more calories than does your body fat. To counter these changes, try to incorporate an exercise program to decrease muscle loss and counter the fact that your body may be burning fewer calories. If you are able to go to a gym, do exercises for all the muscle groups. If you cannot go to a gym, doing push-ups, squats, and sit-ups at home will also help. As mentioned in chapter 2, walking, swimming, and jogging are also important for your heart health.

## Increase Dietary Fiber

A major goal of the Smart Diet for CKD is to get most of your carbohydrates from fruits, vegetables, fat-free and low-fat dairy, and whole grains rather than refined grains. Refined grains are made from whole grains that are processed to make them easier to digest and to have a longer shelf life. This processing removes the health-promoting fiber.

Fiber is a type of carbohydrate that your body cannot digest. Many foods with carbohydrates also supply fiber. Food labels can help you focus on increasing dietary fiber. By increasing fiber in your diet, you help lower cholesterol and blood sugar, reduce your diabetes risk, decrease constipation and other irritable bowel symptoms, and decrease your risk of colon cancer. You get more fiber in your diet by leaving the skins on your fruits and vegetables and by choosing whole fruits over fruit juice.

Most of the foods in an average American diet contain refined grains that are low in fiber, examples of which are bagels, corn bread, muffins, bread crumbs, biscuits, crackers, white breads, pretzels, pizza, cakes, cookies, tortillas, waffles, white rice, and noodles. Try to decrease your intake of these foods. Food labels will tell you how much fiber is in the food. Try to increase whole grains in your diet.

## Decrease Bad Fats and Increase Good Fats

Eating too much saturated fat can increase your LDL. Getting rid of saturated fats should help decrease your atherosclerosis risk, as long as you replace these foods with healthier choices. Some patients reduce their saturated-fat intake but increase their intake of sugars and other carbohydrates. High sugar intake may worsen atherosclerosis. Your best bet is to replace saturated fat with polyunsaturated fat but not with sugars and other carbohydrates. Saturated fats are found in the greatest amounts in lard, butter, shortening, egg yolks, red meat, whole milk, beef fat, coconut and palm oils, fatty meats, dairy, cakes, cookies, and fast foods like pizza, burgers, and tacos. Try to decrease your intake of these foods. Consider using spices in place of butter or fatty ingredients to get more flavor from your food.

Even if you follow a low-fat diet, most CKD patients will require cholesterol medications to get your LDL below 100, or below 70 for diabetics.

## Decrease Sodium

A high salt intake can increase your blood pressure, worsen your symptoms of congestive heart failure, and may play a role in worsening atherosclerosis. Although unproven, a high-salt diet may worsen kidney function. When looking for foods that are low in sodium, be careful with "Lite Salt," which is potassium chloride. As your kidney function decreases, you may need to decrease your potassium intake.

Your total sodium intake should be less than 2,300 mg a day. An average American diet has around 3,400 mg, and many patients eat more than 8,000 mg a day. When you look at food labels to see how much sodium is in an average serving, you will realize that you are eating a lot of sodium!

## Eating the Right Amount of Protein

Proteins are very important. They build and repair tissue, fight infection, and provide energy. Proteins have a complex relationship to CKD, including their effect on the rate of loss of kidney function. (This aspect of proteins will be discussed in chapter 5.) A high-protein diet may not only be harmful to the kidneys, but it may also make the retention of acids with progressive CKD worse. High protein intakes can also worsen two of the challenges of advancing kidney disease: CKD-related bone disease and CKD-related increased blood phosphorus. On the other hand, if you are on a low- and especially a very-low-protein diet that does not include essential proteins, this diet can worsen the malnutrition and loss of body muscle that comes with progressive CKD.

It turns out that the average American eats around 100 grams of protein a day. However, most nutritional organizations recommend a diet allowance for protein of 0.36 grams per pound of your body weight, so if you weigh 200 pounds, that's 72 grams of protein a day; if you weigh 150 pounds, that's 54 grams of protein per day. Therefore, if the average diet contains 100 grams of protein a day, most CKD patients have a ways to go to get to a low-protein diet.

As we will discuss in chapter 5, there may be a benefit of relatively low-protein diets to slow loss of kidney function. With this in mind, a low-protein diet of 0.3 grams diet protein per pound of your weight per day is a reasonable goal. For most patients, I do not recommend a very-low-protein diet, around 0.15 grams protein per pound of body weight. If you weigh 200 pounds, a very-low-protein diet is 30 grams of protein a day, and if you weigh 150 pounds, that's 23 grams of protein a day. As you can see from these examples and when you plug in your own weight, low- or very-low-protein diets will force you to cut way down on the protein you eat.

When you start reading food labels, you will quickly see that it is very difficult to get to these low-protein diet levels. Research studies of low protein and kidney function found that very few patients were willing to undergo the drastic cuts in the amounts of protein they eat.

## Low- and Very-Low-Protein Diets Versus the Smart Diet for CKD

When you consider the diet protein issue, you need to be realistic about how restrictive you are willing to be. In my experience, most patients are not willing to eat only 20 to 30 grams of protein per day on a very-low-protein diet. My emphasis on the Smart Diet for CKD goes beyond its potential to slow loss of kidney function. The Smart Diet may also help you live longer since it is low in added sugars, saturated fat, cholesterol, sodium, and phosphorus and high in fiber.

If you decide to use a low-protein diet, and especially if you choose to go on a very-low-protein diet, you need the support of a licensed dietician to be sure that you are getting enough essential protein components to avoid malnutrition.

## Avoiding Phosphorus

Phosphorus is added to many foods as a preservative and to give color and flavor to food. Added phosphorus is more harmful to you than natural phosphorus in food. Unfortunately, most food labels do not include the phosphorus content of a food. Some food labels show "phos" as an ingredient, which is a food with added phosphorus. These foods should be decreased or eliminated as your kidney function declines. Chapter 8 explains how high blood phosphorus levels can lead to problems with your bones, blood vessels, and heart.

49

# Recommended Foods as Part of the Smart Diet for CKD:

### Proteins

Fat-free or low-fat dairy foods: milk, cheese, yogurt

Fish, which is high in omega-3 fatty acids: salmon, tuna, trout

Lean meats (try to avoid red meats): chicken and turkey, should be skinless

Eggs, good source of a complete protein

Soy products: tofu (soybean curd), food alternatives made with soy (soy bacon, soy cheese, soy ice cream, soy burgers, soy dogs, soy chicken-less nuggets, edamame, soy milk, tempeh—soy meat substitute)

### Vegetables—A Source of Protein and Fiber

Legumes: kidney beans, lentils, chickpeas, black-eyed peas, lima beans

Leafy greens: spinach, collard greens, kale

Cruciferous: broccoli, cabbage

Root vegetables: carrots, yams, beets , turnips

### Nuts and Seeds—Another Source of Protein and Fiber

Walnuts, almonds, pine nuts, sesame seeds, sunflower seeds, pumpkin seeds, flax seeds, nut and seed butters, popcorn

*Fruits*

Apples, bananas, oranges, pears, grapes, prunes

*Unsaturated Fats*

Oils: canola, corn, olive, safflower, sunflower, and soybean

*Whole Grains*

Oatmeal and oat bran, brown rice, whole-grain bread or tortillas, barley, whole wheat

## What to Avoid:

Avoid processed meats such as cold cuts, canned foods, frozen foods, prepared meals and packaged foods; organ meats like liver; dairy products that are not fat free; and bottled beverages, especially sodas.

### Advanced CKD Smart Diet Modifications

With low levels of kidney function, you may need to restrict your potassium intake. A diet that is high in fruits, vegetables, whole grains, and seeds is often very high in potassium. Chapter 7 will discuss potassium management in detail. It provides a list of foods that are high in potassium.

With progressive CKD, increasing blood phosphorus

levels becomes more of a problem. Chapter 8 provides a list of foods that are high in phosphorus. A licensed dietician can help you continue a modified Smart Diet with foods that are lower in potassium and phosphorus.

## Modified Smart Diet for Older Adults with CKD

Currently, there are no specific diet recommendations for older adults with CKD. Chapter 5 will go into detail regarding daily protein intakes to possibly slow the loss of kidney function. For all patients, the potential adverse effects of low-protein diets on overall nutrition are a concern. Older patients are more prone to the progressive decline in overall nutrition that comes with advancing CKD. Muscle loss is a common problem as patients age. This loss may be even faster as patients lose kidney function. The harmful effects of this muscle loss may include an increase in falls, which is one of the biggest health issues for older patients. Older adults should enlist the help of a kidney dietician specialist to be sure that you are getting the right types and amounts of protein to prevent muscle loss and malnutrition.

## Recipes

There are several free recipe books for kidney patients. Go to www.kidney.org to get the US National Kidney Foundation Family Recipe Cookbook. At www.davita.com, you can get kidney-friendly recipes.

## Diet Supplements

The US National Kidney Foundation has a web page devoted to herbal supplements. I highly recommend all patients with CKD read their guide to herbal supplements. Herbal supplements can actually make your kidney disease worse. I understand the desire to find a cure for your kidney problem, but using these supplements is risky and there is no good science to justify their use for CKD. There are very few research studies on these supplements, and even fewer have been studied in patients with CKD. Supplements are not regulated by the FDA and many come from other countries. Supplements are not required to undergo patient safety and efficacy to see if they work and whether they might be harmful.

By contrast, any medication you are prescribed has strict safety and efficacy requirements before the FDA will approve their use. Drug companies have to follow strict guidelines when they manufacture these medicines. Manufacturing of dietary supplements is not regulated. Many supplements have been found to have impurities and often they may contain a mixture of potentially dangerous substances. Also, as opposed to your prescription meds, there is no requirement to report bad effects from these supplements. Some have harmful heavy metals and others aristolochic acid, which has proven harmful for kidneys. These supplements can interact with your prescription medicines and raise or lower their blood levels. Many of them have high amounts of potassium and phosphorus.

There are many "kidney supplements" available online.

None have a proven benefit. I advise you to save your time and money by avoiding these expensive and potentially dangerous products. As we will discuss in chapter 5, very-low-protein diets are rarely indicated for patients with an eGFR over 30 unless you have high levels of urine protein and are losing kidney function rapidly.

## SUMMARY

The Smart Diet for CKD patients can help address obesity, kidney disease progression, hardening of your arteries, retention of acids, diabetes risk, and uncontrolled blood pressure. The diet consists of smaller portion sizes, fewer overall calories, fewer carbohydrates and sugary foods, a lower dietary protein intake, a limit of alcohol intake to one drink per day, more fiber through the intake of more whole grains and fewer refined grains, avoidance of saturated fats and a decrease of sodium and phosphorus intake. I realize the challenges of changing from your current diet to the Smart Diet for CKD. Try to gradually modify your diet so that you don't get overwhelmed. Try some of the free recipes, and happy dining!

# Chapter 4

## Reversible Declines in Kidney Function

ANYONE WITH DECREASED KIDNEY function would love to hear that that their kidney function will get better. Reversible declines in kidney function (also called AKI or acute kidney injury) are one of the most common reasons patients are sent to a kidney specialist. In my experience, many of these drops are just a lab issue. A repeat eGFR will be back to your prior level. Causes of AKI and ways to prevent AKI are reviewed in this chapter. You will also learn about a more serious form of AKI called acute tubular necrosis, or ATN. ATN in many cases leads to dialysis. Recovery of kidney function is always important to look for, even after dialysis has started.

## What Can Lead to a Reversible Drop in Kidney Function?

Temporary drops in kidney function include many different scenarios. These range from things that cause you to become less well hydrated, to the declines in kidney function that may come from a weak heart.

Steven Rosansky

## Dehydration—the Most Common Cause of a Reversible Decline in Kidney Function

If the fluid part of your blood (called plasma) or the red blood cells get too low (for example from bleeding), your kidney function may drop. I will use a fuel tank analogy to help you understand how dehydration works. Let's assume that the fluid and blood cells in your blood vessels are what fills your "tank." If your tank level is too low, you need to refill it. If your kidneys are working well, most of the salt and water that your kidneys filter, the glomerular filtrate (see eGFR, chapter 1) goes back into your bloodstream. This helps to keep your tank full. If you don't take in enough fluids as a result of the flu, or another illness, or if you get severely overheated and sweat a lot, the fluid level in your tank will drop. You can also lower your tank level with vomiting, diarrhea, or after taking too many water pills (diuretics).

To treat your dehydration, some of you may wind up in the hospital to get intravenous (IV) fluids. Even if your kidney function goes way down, it will likely fully recover with patience and attention to getting your tank full again. This is not a reason to start dialysis in most situations.

## Acute Tubular Necrosis-ATN

An exception to these easily reversible scenarios is called ATN, or acute tubular necrosis. ATN is a type of AKI (temporary decline in your kidney function). If you get extremely dehydrated, take too much blood pressure medication, or have some other event that causes your blood pressure to drop below 90 systolic for an extended period, you may get ATN. ATN temporarily shuts the kidneys down. Some patients require dialysis for days to weeks until the ATN reverses.

## The Need to Look for Recovery of Kidney Function After Starting Dialysis

In most cases of ATN, your kidney function will recover. Unfortunately, once dialysis is started, many dialysis providers do not check for recovery of kidney function. If you are a patient who starts dialysis after a large drop in your kidney function, you should ask your kidney doctor if your kidney function has improved enough to get off dialysis! An example of this kidney function recovery was seen with Art Buchwald, a well-known humor columnist. At age eighty-one, Mr. Buchwald had severe worsening of his kidney function. His doctors started dialysis. They told him that he would die within days if he stopped dialysis. Mr. Buchwald was "ready for the end" and took himself off dialysis. To everyone's surprise, he did well for almost one year without dialysis. My educated guess is that Mr. Buchwald had a reversible decline in his kidney function during his hospitalization. He likely had enough kidney function recovery to remain off dialysis.

*Patient Who Recovered Kidney Function and Stopped Dialysis*

Here is an example of a patient of mine who started dialysis after an AKI and was able to come off dialysis. Mr. T presented to me with an eGFR of around 8. He never knew that he had a kidney problem. We dialyzed Mr. T for three weeks. Mr. T noticed that he was making more urine. I decided to stop his dialysis so that we could measure how much kidney function he had. He had an eGFR of around 12. I had Mr. T come to our dialysis unit for blood tests every week for about for a month. His kidney function continued to improve and he remained off dialysis.

## Reversible Drops in eGFR from Medications

Some medications can cause a temporary or even a permanent drop in your kidney function. This is especially common when your "tank" needs filling, i.e., from dehydration. Over-the-counter pain medications, including NSAIDs (nonsteroidal anti-inflammatory drugs) and ACE (angiotensin-converting enzyme inhibitors) and ARB (angiotensin-receptor blockers) drugs are often the culprits.

The NSAIDs can drop eGFR by decreasing the blood flow to the kidneys, especially in patients who are dehydrated, or in patients with heart failure or liver failure. Over-the-counter NSAIDs include Aleve, Motrin, Advil, and Celebrex. The drops in eGFR with NSAIDs can be made worse if you are also taking an ACE or an ARB.

The ACEs and the ARBs are very important drugs for CKD patients. An ACE inhibitor is an angiotensin-converting enzyme inhibitor, which can help relax your veins and arteries to lower your blood pressure. ACE inhibitors prevent an enzyme in your body from producing angiotensin II, a substance that narrows your blood vessels. This narrowing can cause high blood pressure and force your heart to work harder. Angiotensin II also releases hormones that raise your blood pressure.

You can tell if you are getting an ACE if the generic name of the drug you are taking has "pril" at the end of it. For example, lisinopril, captopril, enalapril, benazepril, fosinopril, gamipril, quinapril, perindopril, trandolapril, moexipril. You can tell if you are on an ARB if the generic name of your blood pressure medication ends in "tan" (losartan, irbesartan, candesartan, valsartan, telmisartan, azilsartan, eprosartan).

As we will discuss in chapter 5, the ACE and the ARB drugs are key to slowing loss of kidney function. The main reason to move from a "pril" to a "tan" drug is if you have a cough on an ACE. Be sure to report any cough that starts with taking your ACE. The ACE can increase the cough reflex in about one out of ten patients. It may need to be stopped and your doctor can try an ARB. In my opinion, all ACEs and ARBs are equally good at slowing loss of kidney function.

Unfortunately, these drugs commonly cause reversible declines in eGFR. When you are first started on an ACE or an ARB, your doctor should check for a drop in kidney function. Interestingly, even with an initial drop in your eGFR, continuation of these drugs can delay or may even prevent a future need for dialysis. In chapter 5, I will explain how to handle the drop in eGFR after starting an ACE or an ARB.

One strategy that may help prevent a drop in eGFR from an ACE or an ARB is to try to hold off from taking any other medicines that can also cause a drop in eGFR, like NSAIDs or proton pump inhibitors (PPIs).

There are many medicines that need a dose adjustment if you have CKD. Your doctor should review your medications at each visit. He needs to be sure that you are getting the appropriate dosing of your meds for your eGFR level and that none of your medicines are harming your kidneys.

As your kidney function declines, some drugs that depend on your kidneys for excretion can accumulate. When these drug levels rise, they can cause dangerous side effects. These side effects can be avoided with appropriate medication dosage adjustment. The need to adjust drug doses for your level of kidney function is one reason to be aware that you have CKD.

### *What About the Proton Pump Inhibitors?*

Some of the drugs widely used for gastroesophageal reflux (GERD) are called proton pump inhibitors (PPIs). PPIs include Prevacid (lansoprazole), Prilosec (omeprazole), Nexium (esomeprazole). Although not proven definitively, these drugs may cause AKI and progressive CKD. My advice is to avoid these drugs if you have mild reflux symptoms and CKD. Preferred medications for those who have CKD and reflux include antacids, like Tums or Rolaids. The best ways to decrease long-term reflux symptoms are to eat small meals, drink less alcohol, and lose weight.

## X-ray Contrast

Intravenous x-ray contrast tests ordered by your doctor may temporarily or even permanently worsen your kidney function. This is more likely to occur if you already have abnormal kidney function. In cases like this, your doctor will have to balance the potential risk of a decline in your kidney function due to the contrast agent versus the diagnostic value of the x-ray. One question to ask your doctor: Will the result of the x-ray report change my treatment?

In the past, after an x-ray of the arteries to heart (coronary angiogram), it was not uncommon for patients with CKD, especially diabetics, to develop irreversible kidney failure, which led to dialysis. With the use of newer contrast agents and proper patient preparation before the x-ray, this scenario is now uncommon.

### *The Importance of Staying Well Hydrated to Decrease the Risk of AKI*

A word of advice from the KDIGO is to stay well hydrated if you need to take any of the drugs that can cause a decline in your kidney function. In addition to being well hydrated, if you need to take x-ray contrast, hold any medicines that can drop eGFR, like ACEs, ARBs, and NSAIDs.

## Heart Failure and AKI

Some of you reading this may have a weak heart—congestive heart failure (CHF). This is a common diagnosis for CKD patients since the frequency of CHF increases as eGFR decreases. Around half of all patients with an eGFR of less than 30 can develop CHF. With CHF, your "tank" may be full, but since you have a weak pump (your heart), your kidneys may not be getting enough pressure. With this low pressure, the kidneys retain salt water. This extra salt water causes edema (swelling in your ankles and/or legs). A quick test for too much salt and water in your body is to take your index finger and press it into the skin at your ankle. A small indentation is okay. A deeper indentation may signal that you have too much salt water in your body.

One of the most common situations that can lead to dialysis is worsening of CHF (see chapter 9). To manage heart failure, high-dose diuretics together with ACE or ARB therapy are commonly prescribed. This can lead to "over diuresis"—too much diuretic, and an ACE- or ARB-related AKI, a temporary drop in eGFR. For some patients with CHF, diuretic-related "dehydration" might be necessary to help you breathe more comfortably and avoid dialysis. Unfortunately, the decline in your kidney function in these situations can lead to dialysis. In these cases, dialysis is mainly to treat heart failure–related fluid overload, rather than for a low level of kidney function.

Some experts accept a decline in kidney function, even up to 40 percent, in situations like this, since there may be a long-term survival benefit and a decrease in hospitalizations with the continued use of the ACE or ARB drugs and diuretics. Your kidney doctor and your heart doctor (cardiologist) need to be sure that you are getting the correct treatments to maximize your heart and kidney function. It may be reasonable for some patients to delay dialysis if diuretic and heart failure drug management control your symptoms. Discuss this option with your kidney treatment team.

## Blockage of Urine Flow from Large Prostate or Kidney Stones

Another common situation that can lead to a reversible decline in kidney function is blockage of urine flow caused by a large prostate (benign prostatic hypertrophy—BPH). Here is a typical story.

I have seen numerous older men who come into the hospital with stage 5 CKD (an eGFR of less than 15). As part of a routine evaluation, I have a catheter passed into the bladder to see if there is retention of urine. Many of these patients had more than a quart of urine retained in the bladder. With a catheter in place to drain the bladder, kidney function returns to normal over days to weeks. In most of these cases, the urine that flows out of the urethra is being blocked by an enlarged prostate.

Kidney stones can also cause a reversible drop in eGFR in both men and women. This situation is not very common. Even if one ureter is blocked by a kidney stone (see chapter 1), there may be little change in kidney function. To cause AKI, kidney stones must block both ureters or a kidney stone must be blocking a patient's only functioning kidney. Since most patients have two functioning kidneys, both of these situations are uncommon. Urologists, the surgeons who deal with diseases of the kidney, urethra, and bladder, have many ways to treat urine-flow blockages. Once the blockage is relieved, most patients' kidney function will return to their baseline value.

Urologists can also treat other causes of AKI due to decreased urine flow. They can remove kidney stones, relieve ureter blockage and blockage of the urethra. They can also help diabetics and other patients who have nerve-damage-related bladder-emptying problems.

## SUMMARY

The first thing any kidney doctor should do is look for reversible causes of a decline in your kidney function. The most reversible cause of decline in your eGFR is dehydration. A second often-overlooked cause is that your blood pressure is too low. If blood pressure is very low for an extended period of time, it can lead to a type of reversible decline in kidney function that may require short-term dialysis. A weak heart can lead to a temporary decline in kidney function. In some cases, patients start long-term dialysis when they have an eGFR over 10 and a weak heart. Staying well hydrated and avoiding a combination of drugs that can cause a decline in kidney function are two important strategies to decrease reversible declines in kidney function.

# Chapter 5

## What You Can Do to Slow the Decline of Your Kidney Function

MOST CKD PATIENTS DO not have high levels of urine protein and therefore lose kidney function slowly, if at all, over time. For patients with high urine protein levels, a lower target blood pressure, a high dose of an ACE or an ARB medication, and a very-low-protein diet may all be appropriate courses of action, as we will discuss in this chapter. Many books for CKD patients encourage the use of low- and very-low-protein diets for all patients with CKD, but in my opinion, very-low-protein diets can be dangerous, since they can lead to malnutrition and potentially shorten your survival.

### Multidisciplinary Follow-Up

In many clinics, patients have a kidney treatment team to help manage their CKD. The team can include a nephrologist, an internist, a nurse practitioner, a physician assistant, a dietician, and often a social worker. The social worker may help you with financial and other personal and family issues related to your CKD treatment. Multidisciplinary follow-up basically means that you see these folks in the clinic or doctor's office. This kind of follow-up, and the ease of having everyone in one office, may slow kidney function decline and help you to delay and possibly avoid dialysis.

## The Main Causes of CKD

Regardless of the cause of your CKD, all of the methods to slow progression of CKD that we discuss later in this chapter are generally applicable.

### Diabetic Kidney Disease

Any of you who have diabetes and protein in your urine may have diabetic kidney disease. There are two main types of diabetes: type 1 and type 2. Type 1 diabetes occurs when the insulin-producing cells of the pancreas are damaged and patients are not able to produce normal amounts of insulin. In type 2 diabetes (adult-onset diabetes), the pancreas makes insulin, but it either doesn't produce enough or the body becomes resistant to insulin's effect and needs higher insulin levels to function. The vast majority of diabetic kidney disease is due to type 2 diabetes. Diabetic CKD accounts for about half of the world's patients that go on to dialysis. Diabetes increases atherosclerosis-related problems of large blood vessels as well as damage to the tiny blood vessels of the kidneys—the glomerular capillaries and the tiny blood vessels in the back of the eyes (diabetic retinopathy). The glomeruli in diabetics can become diseased and "leaky" to protein.

The small arteries in the back of the eye can leak and branch, too. These changes can result in loss of vision. It is very important that if you are a diabetic with CKD, you have the back of your eyes examined by an optometrist, the doctor who also fits you for glasses. If you have diabetic retinopathy, an ophthalmologist—an eye surgeon—will treat these abnormal blood vessels. If treated early, blindness can be prevented.

Regarding progression of CKD in diabetics, a new class of drugs to lower blood sugar may also slow loss of kidney function. These SGLT2 inhibitors have names that end in gliflozin, like canagliflozin, dapagliflozin, and empagliflozin. These drugs work by preventing glucose from being absorbed in the kidneys. As a result, they decrease glucose in the blood and cause it to spill into the urine. SGLT2 inhibitors may decrease urine protein and may also slow the decline in kidney function for some patients with an eGFR over 30.

*Hypertension and Kidney Disease—Hypertensive Nephropathy*

Eight out of ten patients who have an eGFR below 60 will have hypertension. The relationship between high blood pressure and kidney disease is a long-standing chicken-and-egg story: High blood pressure can cause kidney damage, and kidney damage itself can cause high blood pressure. The association of high blood pressure and kidney disease is called hypertensive nephropathy.

Although this is usually considered to be one type of kidney disease, it really includes a variety of kidney problems. If you are

African American, kidney disease may run in your family. This inherited type of kidney disease may be a glomerular disease and not hypertensive nephropathy. In most cases, patients who have a long history of high blood pressure without a lot of urine protein are called hypertensive nephropathy. It is unusual for a patient to get a kidney biopsy if they have long-standing high blood pressure without a lot of urine protein. Thus, we really don't know the actual cause of CKD in these situations. African Americans are four times more likely to develop kidney failure and start dialysis compared to non-Hispanic white Americans. The two most common causes of kidney failure in African Americans are diabetic and hypertensive nephropathy.

### *Atherosclerosis (Hardening of the Arteries) as a Cause of CKD*

As we discussed in chapter 2, hardening and narrowing of your arteries can be made worse by CKD. This atherosclerotic process by itself can cause a decrease in eGFR. In older adults with CKD, it is often assumed that declines in eGFR are due to decreased blood flow to the kidneys from progressive atherosclerosis. Patients with this type of kidney disease have small amounts of protein in the urine.

### *Glomerular Diseases*

The hallmark of glomerular disease is high levels of urine protein. The long list of glomerular diseases and their treatment is beyond the scope of this book. As mentioned, patients with diabetic CKD and some patients with hypertensive nephropathy may actually have forms of glomerular disease. Leaving aside these two, glomerular disease accounts for about one in ten patients who go on to dialysis in the developed world. Most glomerular diseases are called "idiopathic," which means we don't know their cause. Lab tests and kidney biopsies are usually done to diagnose the particular form of glomerular disease. Many glomerular diseases do not respond to treatment. Some will respond to drugs that depress the immune system.

For all types of glomerular disease, ACE or ARB therapy should be considered to decrease urine protein and slow the decline of eGFR.

### Polycystic Kidney Disease

Polycystic kidney disease (PCKD) is the most well-known inherited kidney disease. This disease accounts for less than 5 percent of patients who go on to dialysis. Over many decades, the kidneys in patients with PCKD develop very large cysts throughout their kidneys. These cystic kidneys can be felt in the belly and can cause pains in the side and back and blood in the urine.

PCKD is usually associated with low levels of protein in the urine. This may in part explain the slow loss of kidney function in most patients with PCKD. One of the main things to help slow the loss of kidney function for PCKD patients is good blood pressure control.

If you have PCKD, be sure to check your children for this

disease, as they have about a fifty-fifty chance of getting PCKD. PCKD can be diagnosed by X-ray and through genetic testing. The disease can pass down through the generations.

A drug called tolvaptan may help slow the loss of kidney function for some patients with PCKD.

## Factors That Relate to the Speed of Decline in Your Kidney Function

There are many things you can do to try to slow loss of kidney function . We will try to focus on what really works. As you will learn one size will not fit every CKD patient.

### Race

In the United States, the rates of dialysis treatment are 3 to 4 times higher for African Americans and 1.5 to 2 times higher for Hispanic white Americans, compared to non-Hispanic white Americans. Some of this may be genetic and can't be changed, but the good news is that if you are in one of these high-risk groups and you decrease your atherosclerosis risk (see chapter 2), you may also decrease the likelihood that you will need dialysis in the future.

### Blood Pressure Control

Good blood pressure control can help slow the decline of your kidney function. Blood pressure <130/80 mmHg is a reasonable blood pressure target for patients with CKD and low levels of urine protein (1+ or less on dipstick). For patients with CKD and significant amounts of protein in the urine (2+ or greater on urine dipstick) the target blood pressures are lower, around 110–120/70–80 mmHg.

Patients with high urine protein levels generally have a more rapid loss of kidney function compared to patients with lower urine protein levels. A lower target blood pressure may help slow this eGFR decline. The reason that a low target blood pressure (110–20 systolic, top number) is not the goal for everyone is the possibility that too low a blood pressure can decrease the blood flow to the kidneys. For some patients, too low a blood pressure may accelerate the loss of kidney function. If you are a patient who is having a rapid loss of kidney function, the lower target blood pressure may slow this decline. In order to minimize this risk, if you are using the 110–120 systolic blood pressure goal, be sure to check your blood pressure at home, especially if you feel weak or dizzy. My suggestion is to not take your blood pressure medicine dose if your systolic blood pressure is around 100 or less. Discuss this with your kidney team. The reason for this approach is that if your systolic blood pressure gets below the 90–100, it may not only harm your kidneys, but may also damage your heart and your brain. Low blood pressures can lead to chest pain, heart attacks, and strokes.

### Difficult to Control Blood Pressure

If your blood pressure is running above 150 systolic or above 90 diastolic on at least two readings, you probably need additional blood pressure medication. It is not unusual for patients with CKD to require three or more different blood pressure medications in order to achieve your goal blood pressure.

One of the most common reasons for poor blood pressure control is failure to take your blood pressure medications. Most blood pressure meds can be taken just once a day. Try to set a schedule where you take your blood pressure meds the same time every day. I shoot for a once-a-day blood pressure regimen to help simplify treatment. Personally, I take all of my medications at night, before bed. In addition to simplifying blood pressure treatment, nighttime dosing may have other benefits, including possibly better long-term survival.

Other factors that can make blood pressure difficult to control are drinking more than two alcoholic drinks a day, eating too much salt, taking a stimulant type of drug like Adderall, or Ritalin for attention deficit disorder, weight loss, or taking these drugs or cocaine, for recreation. As we discussed in chapter 2, another situation that leads to problems with blood pressure control is "white-coat hypertension," when your blood pressure readings are higher at your doctor's office than at home. If you are not taking a diuretic as part of your blood pressure regimen, this can make your blood pressure difficult to control. Many blood pressure drugs contain a diuretic together with another type of drug. This combination is a good idea. My first choice for treating high blood pressure in CKD patients who have proteinuria is an ACE or an ARB together with a water pill (diuretic).

## Level of Protein in Your Urine

Of all the clinical issues that relate to a faster loss of kidney function, the amount of protein in your urine (proteinuria) may be most important. There is an enormous amount of kidney research on factors that relate to a faster decline of kidney function. Proteinuria comes out to be the most powerful predictor of kidney function loss.

As described in chapter 1, the ballpark amount of protein in your urine can be estimated with a simple urinalysis. More reliable and more specific measures are the "spot" urine protein and the twenty-four-hour urine collections for protein. Since the amount of protein in your urine can be decreased by using an ACE or an ARB, these medications are very important for CKD patients. Some of you may wonder about combining an ACE and an ARB—this is not recommended, since when combined they may decrease your eGFR.

Any patient with CKD who has protein in their urine should be considered for treatment with an ACE or an ARB. If your urine protein runs around 1+, your target blood pressure is around 130 systolic. In this case the ACE or ARB does not have to be given at a high dose.

If you have a significant amount of protein in your urine (more than 300 mg per day, or consistently 2+ or more on dipstick), the combination of either an ACE or an ARB (not both) at the highest dose tolerated, plus a diuretic to get to a goal blood pressure of 110–120/75–79 mmHg may be the best way to decrease progressive hardening of your arteries, decrease the protein in your urine, slow the decline in your kidney function, and decrease the likelihood of dialysis in the future.

### What if an ACE or an ARB Causes a Drop in Your eGFR?

For CKD patients with 1+ protein or less on urinalysis, it is probably best to stop the ACE or ARB if eGFR declines.

If you have more protein on urinalysis, and especially if you have over 300 mg per day of urine protein (called macroalbuminuria), continuing the ACE or ARB may have long-term benefits for your kidney function, despite an initial eGFR decline. With this in mind, many kidney experts suggest continuing these drugs even after a 30 percent decrease in eGFR. If you are one of these patients, you should discuss your treatment options with your kidney team.

## Patient Example

*A Patient with a Reversible Decline in Kidney Function from ACE/ARB Therapy*

Here is an example of how an ACE or an ARB can cause a short-term change in eGFR. Mr. P. is a fifty-year-old male with a long-standing history of hypertension. He had more than 300 mg protein in his urine. After starting losartan (an ARB), his kidney function showed a decline. I discussed the possibility that this short-term change may reverse and that the losartan was an important drug for him to take. Sure enough, over the next six months his kidney function returned to his baseline, and he has been stable for four years on losartan.

## Low- and Very-Low-Protein Diets to Slow Loss of Kidney Function

The topic of low-protein diets and their effect on your kidney function has been a hotly debated topic among kidney specialists since the first randomized controlled trial on the issue was published in 1994. When all the published studies are put together, there seems to be some benefit of low-protein diets to slow decline of renal function. The benefit for diabetics is less clear than for nondiabetics.

## Low-Protein Diet Not Recommended for Diabetics with CKD

The most recent proposal by KDIGO for diabetics with CKD who are not on dialysis is 0.36 mg protein per pound of body weight per day. This is just a bit higher than the protein intake of my Smart Diet for CKD. KDIGO experts feel that diabetics already restrict carbohydrates, fats, and alcohol. Restricting protein on top of these diet restrictions can have adverse impacts on a diabetic patient's quality of life and may cause undesired weight loss and malnutrition. Also, adequate protein intake in diabetics with CKD is important to help prevent dangerously low blood sugars.

## Low-Protein Diets for Nondiabetic CKD Patients

Most of the studies on low-protein diets looked at patients with more advanced stages of CKD—mostly stage 4 and 5 CKD, with an eGFR below 30. After reviewing the recommendations of KDI-GO and research papers on low- and very-low-protein diets, here is my conclusion: It is unlikely that patients with eGFRs in the 45+ range, without large amounts of urine protein, will ever face dialysis. Thus, for most patients with CKD, I do not recommend very-low-protein diets, with or without keto-acid supplements. I feel that the enormous effort to achieve a very-low-protein intake and the high cost of the diet supplements that are prescribed with this diet are not justified for the vast majority of patients with CKD. If you have urine protein levels consistently of 2+ or more, or if there is evidence that your kidney function is declining quickly, a very-low-protein diet can be considered. A fast rate of decline is a loss of more than five units of eGFR per year (see chapter 6).

I encourage a relatively low-in-protein intake as part of my Smart Diet for CKD. To me there is no need for a drastic reduction in dietary protein for most patients. The Smart Diet for CKD has many life-prolonging benefits in addition to its benefit for kidney function.

Patients who are convinced that they want to follow a very-low-protein diet must consider malnutrition. As your kidney function declines, your overall nutrition may also get worse. Older patients may need higher dietary protein intakes to prevent progressive loss of body muscle. In a twenty-year study, women with a higher protein intake had fewer falls, fewer fractures, and a better ability to walk. When I consider the slow decline of kidney function in older patients and the need to maintain a good nutritional state, I do not recommend low- or very-low-protein diets for older folks with CKD.

### When to Consider A Very Low Protein Diet

If you are a patient who has high levels of urine protein and therefore are expected to lose kidney function rapidly, a very-low-protein diet might make sense. High levels of urine protein means a spot urine protein of 300 or more and a dipstick urine protein of 2+ or more. By reducing protein intake, you can also decrease the acidosis that comes with progressive CKD. Decreasing acidosis by itself may decrease the rate of kidney function loss. If you decide to go on a very-low-protein diet, consult your renal team's dietician to be sure you are getting adequate calories and the essential proteins in your diet.

There is a good randomized controlled study comparing low- and very-low-protein diets for nondiabetic patients, some with an eGFR of less than 30 and some with an eGFR of less than 20. The patients on the very-low-protein diet also got ketoanalogues, a pill that helps provide the essential components of proteins to prevent malnutrition.

Only about 15 percent of the patients who initially signed up for the study were willing and able to follow the low–protein diets. Nevertheless, for very motivated nondiabetic patients with urine protein levels of 2+ or more and with eGFRs less than 30, a very-low-protein diet with ketoanalogue supplements may be reasonable. This approach is expensive and very difficult to follow for most patients. If your eGFR is over 40 and you do not have high levels of urine protein, I recommend that you stick to the Smart Diet for CKD.

## Very-Low-Protein Diets with Keto-Acid Supplements for Patients Who Choose Non-Dialysis Management

The very-low-protein diet with keto-acid supplements can also be used to decrease the symptoms of kidney failure. If your kidney function declines to very low levels (an eGFR around 5) and your family has decided against chronic dialysis, very-low-protein diets with keto-acid supplements should be considered to decrease symptoms of kidney failure.

## Blood Sugar Control

Most patients assume that keeping blood sugar in a normal range will slow the decline of kidney function and help you to live longer. This may not be correct.

If you are a type 1 or type 2 diabetic who does not have CKD, keeping your A1C in the 6 to 7 range can prevent you from getting chronic kidney disease. But if you are a diabetic who already has CKD, there is no convincing evidence that keeping blood sugars close to normal and keeping your A1C below 7 can slow the loss of your kidney function. CKD patients who try to get their A1C below 7 can increase their likelihood of getting dangerously low blood sugars. CKD increases the risk of hypoglycemia (low blood sugar). The risk of hypoglycemia is greatest for diabetics with CKD, where the goal of an A1C of 7 to 8 may be a safe approach. Patients who have had a stroke or a heart attack and older patients with a limited life expectancy can shoot for an A1C in the 8 range (see chapter 2).

## Alkali Therapy

If you have an eGFR below 30, you may have too much acid and not enough alkali in your blood. Some research studies suggest that if you raise your blood alkali, you may slow the loss of your kidney function (see chapter7). Alkali refers to something you probably already have in your kitchen—baking soda, which is technically sodium bicarbonate. If you take sodium bicarbonate or another form of alkali, it may not only slow your kidney function loss, but this might also decrease the breakdown of muscle proteins that occurs with low levels of kidney function. A note of caution: If you have heart failure, the sodium load from sodium bicarbonate pills can worsen your heart condition. Discuss this with your kidney team.

I strongly suggest all CKD patients try to follow the Smart Diet for CKD that I described in chapter 3. This diet will produce less acid. If you have a blood bicarbonate of less than 22 (see chapter 8), adding baking soda to the Smart Diet for CKD may help slow the loss of your kidney function.

## Should You Drink a Lot of Water to Slow Loss of Kidney Function?

As I mentioned in chapter 3, drinking a lot of water might help some patients lose weight. Regarding loss of kidney function, however, the only randomized controlled study that looked at this issue was done by my colleague Dr. W. Clark. Although this study did not show a benefit in the loss of eGFR from drinking large amounts of water, it did slow the decline of creatinine clearance (see chapter 1). In other words, the study was not conclusive. In general, patients need to take in as much water as they lose. Some of this water loss is called insensible. This means that the water loss is not noticed. This water loss can be in sweat or in your breath. Although drinking a lot of water may not slow the decline in kidney function, it is important to take in enough fluids to avoid dehydration. If you are having fevers, excessive sweating from work or the heat, you need to replenish your body water to prevent a decline in your kidney function. Also, as we discussed in chapter 4, if you are taking any of the drugs that can drop your eGFR, like ACEs, ARBs, or NSAIDs, you need to stay well hydrated to protect your kidneys.

For patients with very low levels of kidney function and patients with advanced heart failure, your kidneys may not get rid of extra fluids. In some of these situations you may need to decrease water intake to prevent water overload.

For most people with CKD, my advice is to just let your thirst be your guide for how much water to drink. The one exception is for patients with kidney stones who may need around two quarts of fluids per day to decrease new stone formation.

## Is it Okay to Use Pain Relievers if You Have CKD?

Many clinicians fear giving their patients with CKD NSAIDs because of their association with a decreased eGFR. It is true that patients with CKD should avoid pain relievers that contain mixtures of aspirin, acetaminophen, and caffeine in one pill, because there is some evidence that very high doses of these mixtures of drugs taken over many years can cause kidney failure.

The major kidney doctor organizations discourage the use of NSAIDs in patients with CKD. The blanket rejection of short-acting over-the-counter NSAIDs for patients with early-stage CKD is not logical. In my opinion and in the opinion of other kidney experts, short-term use of these drugs at the recommended doses for a patient with an eGFR over 30 may be fine. On the other hand, patients with advanced stages of CKD may be at higher risk of a decline in eGFR or a rise in blood potassium levels with NSAID use. Older patients may be at higher risk of bleeding in the stomach from NSAIDs. Use of short-acting NSAIDs (ibuprofen, Motrin) at the recommended dosage on the pill bottle, for short periods, in patients under sixty year of age, with an eGFR over 30 or so, should be fine. It is a good idea to get used to reading the labels of any over-the-counter pain relievers to see the recommended doses and if the pain reliever contains multiple ingredients. Although not proven to cause kidney failure, it is wise to avoid the long-term use of high doses of single-ingredient NSAIDs, like ibuprofen (Motrin), naproxen (Aleve), and even aspirin.

Alternative pain medicine that will not hurt your kidneys include topical NSAIDs and acetaminophen. The use of topical NSAID patches, gels, sprays, and creams, like diclofenac (Voltaren), ibuprofen (Nurofen), ketoprofen (Orudis), indomethacin (Indocin), and piroxicam (Feldene) will not hurt the kidneys and can provide the same pain relief as NSAIDs taken by mouth. A typical brand of acetaminophen is Tylenol, but there are many others. You can take up to a max dose of two 500 mg tabs of acetaminophen four times a day.

There is a lot of controversy over the use of opiates. A low-dose opiate in combination with acetaminophen may be an appropriate pain treatment alternative for some patients.

## What About Aspirin to Prevent Heart Attack or Stroke?

The regular use of aspirin in the small doses recommended for the prevention of heart attack or stroke will not hurt your kidneys. Use of a baby aspirin (81–162 mg daily) is probably fine, even if you have reduced kidney function. Recent reports emphasize benefits of a baby aspirin after a heart attack or a stroke to prevent a recurrence. On the other hand, for patients who have not had a heart attack or a stroke, use of a baby aspirin to prevent one of these outcomes (so-called primary prevention) is controversial. Daily use of a baby aspirin is associated with an increased bleeding risk. This increased risk of having a bleed in the brain or stomach may outweigh the benefit of low-dose aspirin in patients that have not had a heart attack or a stroke. Discuss this with your kidney treatment team.

### SUMMARY

Although everyone who deals with kidney disease would love to find a new magic bullet to slow kidney function loss, there are only two types of drugs that have consistently proven beneficial, and these are the ACE and ARB drugs. These drugs are especially important if you have lots of protein in your urine and therefore are at a higher risk of losing kidney function rapidly. Many of the suggestions to slow hardening of your arteries given in chapter 2, like blood pressure control and a diet high in fruits and vegetables, may not only help you live longer but may also slow the loss of your kidney function. As part of your lifestyle changes, my Smart Diet for CKD is worth considering. This diet will not only lower your atherosclerosis risk, but it may also slow the loss of your kidney function and decrease muscle breakdown and acidosis that can come with lower levels of kidney function. Patients with high levels of urine protein should consider a lower target for your blood pressure (110–120 systolic) the maximum-tolerated dose of an ACE or an ARB, and sodium bicarbonate if your blood bicarbonate is less than 22. Nondiabetic patients with high levels of urine protein and an eGFR less than 30 may want to consider a very-low-protein diet with or without keto-acid supplements. A very low protein diet approach does not make sense for the vast majority of CKD patients and requires the help of a licensed dietician to avoid malnutrition. The lifestyle changes of chapter 2 and the Smart Diet for CKD, chapter 3, are appropriate for all CKD patients. If your kidney function has declined to an eGFR in the 30 or below range and your kidney doctor has ruled out reversible drops in kidney function, it is time to consider the possibility of dialysis in your future. The next chapter will help you predict the likelihood that you will need dialysis.

# PART 2

# KEEPING HEALTHY AS LONG AS POSSIBLE WITHOUT DIALYSIS

IN THIS SECTION OF the book I will explain how to safely delay the start of dialysis. For the vast majority of patients with early-stage CKD, a dialysis decision will not be necessary.

I will help you to get a better idea of whether you are even likely to need dialysis. Chapter 6 provides several ways to determine if a dialysis decision will be needed. These methods require assistance from your kidney treatment team. For some of you, delaying dialysis may mean never starting dialysis. I will explain why.

As part of my effort to maximize your time off dialysis and to keep you as healthy as possible for as long as possible, I explain the recommended treatments for medical conditions associated with advanced CKD. By advanced CKD, I refer to patients with an eGFR in the 30 or below range.

Chapter 7 focuses on the most common and important fluid, electrolyte, and acid base problems that you may face. The chapter focuses on two of the electrolytes, potassium and bicarbonate. A key goal is to be sure that your blood potassium does not get to a life-threatening level. Next, I review how to keep acids from building up in your blood. I finish the chapter with a discussion of diuretics. Diuretics are very commonly used in patients with advanced CKD. Diuretics can change your body fluids and electrolytes. To stay healthy, you need to maintain a balance of your fluids and electrolytes. I describe the fluid and electrolyte problems that can justify the need for starting dialysis.

In chapter 8, we discuss anemia and bone disease associated with progressive CKD. I review the best ways to diagnose and treat these advanced CKD issues.

# Chapter 6

## A Look into the Crystal Ball: How Likely Is It that You Will Need Dialysis in the Future?

THE MAIN GOAL OF this chapter is to understand the factors that relate to whether you will need dialysis. There are four main issues. The first issue is how long you are expected to live. No one lives forever. Certainly, if you are a young patient with CKD 4 or 5 (eGFR less than 30), the likelihood of needing dialysis before you die is very high. On the other hand, if you're in your eighties or nineties, with the same eGFR, you are much less likely to need dialysis in your lifetime. The second issue is how fast your kidney function is declining. This best predictor of a rapid decline is a large amount of protein in your urine. A third factor is how long the start of dialysis can be delayed. The last and least predictable issue is whether you develop an AKI, a large short-term drop in your kidney function. Because of this last issue, there is no way to be certain about who will need dialysis. Nevertheless, if you use the methods that I describe in this chapter, you will get a pretty good idea of whether you are very likely or very unlikely to need dialysis in the future.

# Factors that Predict a Future Dialysis Need

## Rate of Loss of Kidney Function

One of the key issues to determine if your CKD  is likely to lead to a need for dialysis or kidney transplant is how quickly, if at all , you are losing kidney function.

### Age and Decline in eGFR

Many patients have stable kidney function for years. This is especially common for CKD patients seventy years of age and older. In one study, more than one in four older patients with an eGFR of 30–60 had stable kidney function for ten years. In another study, one in three older patients with eGFRs below 30 had a stable kidney function for two years. Several studies have shown that the likelihood of going on dialysis decreases with increasing age. For older patients with an eGFR below 30 (CKD 4 and 5), dialysis is much less likely compared to younger patients with the same eGFR.

Clearly, your age will play a big part in whether you will need dialysis. There are two reasons for this. Older patients tend to lose kidney function more slowly than younger patients. As you know by now, a high urine protein level predicts a faster loss of kidney function, and older patients are unlikely to have high levels of protein in their urine compared to younger patients. A second reason is that older patients are not expected to survive as long as younger patients. This sets up a competition of sorts between when dialysis is needed and when a patient dies from some other cause besides kidney failure.

The normal rate of loss of kidney function is around one unit of eGFR per year. If you lose less than two units per year, you have a pretty slow loss of kidney function. If you lose three to five units per year, you are losing kidney function a little fast. If your eGFR is going down by more than five units per year, you have a rapid loss of kidney function. Most of the patients who go on to dialysis lose their kidney function at a rate greater than five units per year. One study found that the rate of eGFR loss the year prior to dialysis varied with age. Patients over eighty lost only three units of eGFR per year, while patients less than sixty years old lost eGFR at a rate of nine units per year in the year prior to starting dialysis.

### Plotting Your eGFR Change Over Time

As we discussed in chapter 1, I encourage you to plot your eGFR results with your kidney team. It is not unusual to see eGFR values bounce around a lot. Nevertheless, when you look at all your eGFR results, you can get an idea of the average amount of eGFR you are losing per year. For example, if your eGFR went from 60 to 30 in the past six years, you are losing an average of five units of eGFR per year (eGFR 60 - eGFR 30 = 30 units of eGFR/6 years = 5 units eGFR loss per year).

If it went from 30 to 15 in the past three years, you are losing about five units of eGFR per year (eGFR 30 - eGFR 15 = 15 units of eGFR/3years = 5 units eGFR loss per year).

## Early or Late Start of Dialysis and Predicting Your Future Dialysis Needs

Let's assume that you have an eGFR around 30 and you are losing five units of eGFR per year. Now let's see how early or late start of dialysis affects the amount of time you have before you start dialysis. If you start dialysis at an eGFR of 15, you will have three years before you start (5 units eGFR loss per year x 3 years = 15units of eGFR loss from a 30 eGFR = 15 eGFR). If your kidney treatment team agrees to start dialysis at eGFR of 5, you would start dialysis in five years. (30 eGFR - loss of 5 units eGFR x 5 years = 25 units, 30 - 25 = 5). So, in this example, a late start of dialysis gives you two years free of the burden of dialysis.

## AKI and Dialysis

For most patients with CKD stages 1, 2, or 3, dialysis is an unlikely outcome. An exception is if you have an AKI episode—a large short-term drop in your eGFR. The prior recorded eGFR for some patients who start dialysis after an AKI episode might be over 30 and even over 60. In some of these situations you may be too sick to make your own decision about starting dialysis. If you are an older patient, you may want to let your family and your kidney treatment team know whether you want dialysis in these AKI situations. For all patients who start dialysis after an AKI, there is a key issue to keep in mind. You should ask your kidney team to check for recovery of your kidney function. It is unclear how many patients who are on long-term dialysis had an eGFR above 30 or above 60, then had an AKI episode and went on dialysis. My best guess is that less than one in ten patients who go on to lifelong dialysis had an eGFR above 30 or above 60 before they started chronic dialysis.

## The Kidney Failure Risk Equation

Another method of predicting whether you will need dialysis is to use the kidney failure risk equation (KFRE). Ask your renal team to help you apply your particular information to this equation. You can find the equation by going to the website www.kidneyfailurerisk.com. KFRE will give you a good idea about whether you will need dialysis in the next two to five years. Urine protein is the most important variable in the KFRE risk equation, since the level of urine protein predicts a faster loss of kidney function.

Here are a couple of examples using KFRE.

### Patient Example 1

Sarah is a seventy-year-old female. Her eGFR is 20 and her urine protein is low, only 30. Sarah has only a seventeen out of a one hundred chance of needing dialysis in the next five years.

**Patient Example 2**

Molly is a seventy-year-old female with an eGFR of 2, but much higher urine protein, 300. Molly is more than twice as likely as Sarah to need dialysis in the next five years—roughly a one in three chance.

One problem I have with this calculator is that it does not consider the probability of dying from some other cause before you ever need dialysis.

## Risk of Dialysis Versus Risk of Death in Patients with eGFR Below 30

There is a more complicated online tool that may be especially useful for older patients. This tool is called Timing of Clinical Outcomes in CKD with Severely Decreased GFR. This application can be found online at ckdpcrisk.org. It shows how urine protein levels will not only affect your future need for dialysis but will also affect your likelihood of dying before you need dialysis. It shows that your chance of needing dialysis before you die from another cause goes down progressively with increasing age.

To use this calculator, you need your age, sex, race, eGFR, your systolic blood pressure, whether you have had any heart problems or diabetes, your urine protein, and whether you are a smoker.

This calculator will give you your two- and four-year risk

of needing dialysis and the likelihood of dying of a non-kidney-failure issue before you need to start dialysis.

Here are two examples.

### Patient Example 1

Jane is a seventy-year-old white female with an eGFR of 20, a systolic blood pressure of 140, no history of cardiovascular disease, no diabetes, urine albumin to creatinine of 30, and not a smoker. This patient is roughly twice as likely to die in the next four years as to go on dialysis (death 21 percent, dialysis 12 percent).

### Patient Example 2

Mary is also a seventy-year-old with an eGFR of 20, a systolic blood pressure of 140, no history of cardiovascular disease, no diabetes, not a smoker, but she has a spot urine protein of 500. In four years, Mary has about a one in four chance of either dying or going on dialysis.

If Mary were eighty years old, in four years she would have a much higher chance of death before she needed dialysis (death around 43 percent, dialysis around 20 percent).

These examples show how proteinuria is a powerful predictor of both death and dialysis and how older age makes dialysis a much less likely future concern.

Both this predictor and KFRE predictor come from populations of patients, many of whom may have started dialysis early. If your dialysis start is delayed, the likelihood of you starting dialysis may be even lower than predicted by these online tools.

## SUMMARY

I encourage you to plot your eGFR data to see if it is stable. If your eGFR is declining over time, get an idea of how fast it is dropping to help you determine a future dialysis need. Use the KFRE predictor with your kidney team to get a better idea of whether you will need dialysis.

Older patients are likely to have a slow rate of kidney function decline. With increasing age, you are more likely to die of a non-kidney-failure issue before you need dialysis. If your eGFR is below 30, I recommend that you get your kidney team to use the competitive risk of death or dialysis calculator at www. ckdpcrisk.org. Since an AKI episode preceding dialysis is hard to predict, discuss what you would like your family to do if a dialysis decision comes up and you are unable to make your own decision.

# Chapter 7

## Electrolyte and Diuretic Management in Advanced CKD

IT'S IMPORTANT TO UNDERSTAND the electrolyte report that comes with the measure of your creatinine and eGFR. This ties in with advanced CKD issues. The main CKD-related issues are high potassium, called hyperkalemia, and increased acid in the blood, termed acidosis. Resistant hyperkalemia is one reason to start dialysis. Proper management of elevated potassium can help delay dialysis. A low serum bicarbonate, part of the electrolyte report, connects to acidosis, which is common with progressive CKD.

We'll discuss diuretic treatments for advanced CKD, how to safely and effectively use diuretics, and how to prevent diuretic-related electrolyte abnormalities.

## The Electrolyte Report

An electrolyte is a substance that conducts electricity when dissolved in water. The electrolyte report includes measures of sodium, potassium, chloride, bicarbonate, and calcium. In this chapter, we'll focus on high and low levels of potassium and bicarbonate. In the next chapter, we'll focus on calcium.

The bicarbonate connects to carbon dioxide ($CO_2$), the gas you breathe out. $CO_2$ is a waste product that is produced when your body breaks down the food you eat. $CO_2$ takes the form of bicarbonate in your blood. The bicarbonate in your blood keeps your blood at the right pH—not too high, which is called alkalotic, or too low, which is called acidotic.

### Alkalosis and Acidosis

The normal range of your blood pH is from 7.35 to 7.45. A level below 7.35 is called acidosis, a level above 7.45 is called alkalosis. There are two types of acidosis and alkalosis. One type, called metabolic, depends on the functioning of the kidney; the other type, respiratory, is influenced by your breathing.

When you breathe in and out, you take in oxygen and blow out carbon dioxide. With advanced lung disease, patients can't blow off enough carbon dioxide. The carbon dioxide that builds up in the blood is an acid substance, so these patients can get respiratory acidosis. Respiratory alkalosis is produced when people have panic attacks and in other high-anxiety situations that result in rapid breathing. Rapid breathing drops $CO_2$ to a low level, which causes respiratory alkalosis.

### *Metabolic Acidosis*

One of the kidneys' jobs is to remove acid from the blood and excrete the acid in your urine. This keeps the blood acid levels from getting too high. When your eGFR drops below 30, your kidneys may no longer be able to get rid of enough acid. This can lead to metabolic acidosis. The buildup of blood acids can cause a loss of bone, a condition called osteoporosis. Osteoporosis increases your chances of fracturing bones like your hips and backbone. Metabolic acidosis can also decrease blood albumin levels. When albumin, an important protein, drops with metabolic acidosis, you can get muscle loss, also called muscle wasting. Correction of acidosis can help slow the drop in blood albumin and possibly slow loss of kidney function. Metabolic acidosis can also affect your blood sugar levels. It can cause your body to build a resistance to insulin. The insulin resistance that comes with CKD-related acidosis can increase atherosclerosis-related problems. Finally, metabolic acidosis is associated with elevated potassium levels in patients with advanced CKD.

### How to Treat Metabolic Acidosis

The Smart Diet for CKD patients (see chapter 3) can have several benefits. In addition to its potential to slow eGFR loss, decreasing meat intake and increasing the fruits and vegetables in your diet (low-protein diet) and decreasing atherosclerosis may also decrease metabolic acidosis.

Try to keep your bicarbonate above 22. If your bicarbonate is still low while eating a low-protein diet, you may need to take sodium bicarbonate tablets or baking soda. Sodium bicarbonate can cause carbon dioxide to form in your stomach and give you gas pains. It can worsen high blood pressure and increase volume overload, which can worsen heart failure. The high-sodium intake from the sodium bicarbonate can be reversed with a low-sodium diet, or with diuretics to get rid of sodium. The gas pains may be decreased by using baking soda versus taking sodium bicarbonate pills.

### Metabolic Alkalosis

Another issue related to blood pH is metabolic alkalosis. The kidneys regulate blood bicarbonate levels to prevent alkalosis as well as acidosis. Metabolic alkalosis occurs when the bicarbonate on your electrolyte report is 28 or more and your breathing rate is normal.

Most advanced CKD patients are on diuretics. Diuretics can cause metabolic alkalosis. Vomiting can also cause metabolic alkalosis. Both of these situations produce a low chloride and an elevated bicarbonate on the electrolyte panel. If you have a decrease in your blood volume from vomiting, you need to have chloride and sodium replaced. To do this, you will receive a sodium chloride/saline solution in your veins from an IV. If you have metabolic alkalosis due to potassium and chloride loss from diuretic therapy, your doctor may give you potassium chloride tablets. If you take potassium tablets to treat metabolic alkalosis or other causes of low potassium, you will need to have your potassium checked regularly to prevent hyperkalemia, which is high potassium. This may require weekly or monthly follow-up of potassium levels.

*Elevated Potassium—Hyperkalemia*

More than half the patients who go on dialysis develop hyperkalemia at some time before they start dialysis. Diabetics are more prone to this problem than are nondiabetics. If your potassium becomes elevated over the course of weeks to months, we call this chronic hyperkalemia. For some patients, having repeated elevated potassium levels may justify starting dialysis. Before I would consider dialysis for chronic hyperkalemia, though, there are a few things I would consider.

First, let's consider why potassium can become a problem with advanced CKD. The reason is simple: The kidneys are the main organs responsible for keeping your blood potassium in a normal range. When kidneys function normally, they are able to get rid of the potassium you eat. When your eGFR drops below 30, your kidneys may not be able to get excrete enough potassium to keep potassium levels in a normal range, which is between 3.6 to 5.2. A level between 5.2 and 6 is considered mild hyperkalemia, and potassium above 6 is more concerning.

High levels and low levels of potassium interfere with the normal electrical circuits in the heart and your muscles. This can lead to muscle weakness, as well as a sensation of tingling, numbness, or burning in your hands, feet, arms, or legs. The most serious electrical issue is the effect of high potassium on your heart (usually over 7), which can show up on your electrocardiogram (EKG) as an irregular heart rhythm. This irregular rhythm can cause the heart to stop working. The most dangerous situation happens when potassium levels rise very quickly. If this occurs, you will need emergency treatment in the hospital. A rise in blood potassium usually comes without symptoms. Your job as an advanced CKD patient is to try to prevent dangerously high potassium levels. To do this, you first need to know what can cause hyperkalemia. An ounce of prevention here can actually save your life. Proper handling of the potassium issue can also help you delay dialysis.

### Lite Salt, Potassium-Sparing Diuretics, and Other Drugs that Can Cause Elevated Potassium

There are several common situations where your potassium might be elevated. Many CKD and heart failure patients are put on a low-salt diet. As a part of this diet, many patients use Lite Salt, which has both sodium and potassium chloride. Most patients who use Lite Salt are not aware that it has a lot of potassium. Another source of ingested potassium is the potassium supplements (potassium chloride) that are often given with diuretics. Most diuretics increase potassium loss. Some diuretics are called potassium-sparing diuretics. These drugs act to block potassium excretion. They are commonly used with other diuretics to prevent a low potassium level. If your doctor prescribes one of the potassium-sparing diuretics, a check on your potassium within a few weeks after starting one of these meds can avoid a dangerously high potassium. Some of these potassium-sparing medications include spironolactone (Aldactone), triamterene (Dyrenium), amiloride (Midamor), eplerenone (Inspra).

Other drugs that are connected to a risk of high potassium

include NSAIDs, sulfamethoxazole and trimethoprim (Bactrim), propranolol, labetalol, and heparin.

### ACE and ARB Therapy and Elevated Potassium

Now for the really tricky but important stuff. As you may recall, there are two classes of medicines that can slow loss of eGFR: ACEs and ARBs. These medicines can also cause hyperkalemia. As a reminder, ACEs have names that end in "pril" (quinapril, lisinopril, benazepril, enalapril, fosinopril, trandolapril, and moexipril). ARBs have a name that ends in "tan" (losartan, irbesartan, candesartan, valsartan, telmisartan, azilsartan, eprosartan). I recommend that anyone with CKD who takes an ACE or an ARB should also take a diuretic to increase urine potassium excretion. This can help decrease your risk of hyperkalemia.

Combination pills also make blood pressure easier to control. These combination pills usually contain the diuretic hydrochlorothiazide (HCTZ) together with an ACE or an ARB. If you are still having problems with your potassium, a more powerful diuretic called a loop diuretic (see below) may help excrete more potassium.

In addition to treating the metabolic acidosis of CKD, sodium bicarbonate can lower potassium. It does this by moving potassium out of the blood and into your cells. Thus, diuretics and bicarbonate can decrease the elevated potassium that may come from ACE or ARB therapy.

### Low-Potassium Diets

Many CKD patients are put on a low-potassium diet as the first line of treatment for elevated potassium. In my opinion, this diet may become necessary only when your potassium remains elevated after correcting the issues we just discussed. Be sure you have stopped the Lite Salt (potassium chloride), potassium pills, and any unnecessary drugs that can raise your potassium (like potassium-sparing diuretics). Be sure you are taking a diuretic and sodium bicarb if these drugs are appropriate. All of these issues need to be discussed with your kidney team. If your potassium remains elevated, your kidney team should consider a low-potassium diet.

Almost all foods have some potassium. The size of the serving you eat (see the food label) is very important. A large serving of a low-potassium food can turn into a high-potassium meal.

Here are a couple of techniques that can decrease the potassium in your foods. If you only have canned goods on hand to eat, be sure to drain the juice in the can and discard it. You should also rinse the canned food with water and drain out the rinse water. For instance, canned beans are full of potassium, so it's important to drain the liquid they are canned in and rinse the beans well in fresh water.

Another thing you can do is called leaching. Leaching is a process by which some potassium can be pulled out of the vegetables you cook. You can wash, peel, cut up, and soak potatoes and vegetables in a large pot of water for two hours before you cook them. Get rid of this water before you start cooking. Cook the potatoes or vegetables in a large pot of water. Consider using low-potassium fruits and vegetables in your cooking.

### Low-Potassium Vegetables:

| | | |
|---|---|---|
| alfalfa | corn | peppers |
| asparagus | cucumber | radish |
| broccoli | eggplant | sprouts, raw, or |
| cabbage | green beans | cooked from frozen |
| cauliflower | kale | yellow squash |
| celery | lettuce | zucchini |
| cooked carrots | peas | |

### Low-Potassium Fruits:

| | | |
|---|---|---|
| apples | peaches | strawberries |
| blackberries | pears | tangerines |
| blueberries | pineapple | watermelon |
| cranberries | plums | |
| grapefruit | raspberries | |

Remember that if you eat a lot of any of these fruits or vegetables at one time, it can become a high-potassium meal.

In addition to using low-potassium fruits and vegetables, you should try to avoid high-potassium foods.

Steven Rosansky

*High-Potassium Fruits:*

| | |
|---|---|
| apricots | nectarines |
| bananas | oranges and orange juice |
| cantaloupe | papaya |
| dried fruit | pomegranate and pomegranate juice |
| honeydew | prune and prune juice |
| kiwi | pumpkin |
| mango | raisins |

*High-Potassium Vegetables:*

| | | |
|---|---|---|
| baked beans | fried onions | potatoes |
| beets | lentils | sweet potatoes |
| broccoli, cooked | okra | tomato paste |
| brussels sprouts | parsnips | tomato sauce |

*Other High-Potassium Foods:*

| | | |
|---|---|---|
| bran products | French fries | seeds |
| chips | granola | tofu |
| chocolate | nuts | whole-wheat products |
| coconut | peanut butter | |

### Low-Potassium Diet versus Smart Diet for CKD

As you can see from the list of foods on a low-potassium diet, many of the foods that are encouraged as part of the Smart Diet for CKD patients will be restricted on the low-potassium diet. A low-potassium diet excludes a lot of fruits, vegetables, and foods high in fiber and whole grains. Before moving away from the Smart Diet for CKD, be sure that your elevated potassium is not caused by your medications or diet supplements.

### Resistant Hyperkalemia

If you have stopped the medicines and dietary supplements that can raise your potassium, have tried diuretics, sodium bicarbonate, and a low-potassium diet, the next step to consider is a potassium-binding medication. I have been able to delay dialysis for many of my patients by using potassium binders. These potassium binders bind the potassium in the gut and pass it out in your stool.

There are some challenges in using this therapy. Potassium binders need to be taken two or three hours before your other medications. The reason to take them separately is that potassium binders can bind to other medications. I have prescribed the original potassium binder, (sodium polystyrene) Kayexalate for more than forty years. Many of my patients were able to keep their potassium under control with once-daily Kayexalate. In rare cases, Kayexalate has been linked to damage to the gut, but I have never seen this in my patients. This rare side effect led to the promotion of two new meds to treat high potassium—patiromer (Veltassa) and sodium zirconium (Lokelma). My guess is that with three drugs to choose from, potassium binders may become a standard way to delay dialysis. Any one of these potassium binders can help keep your potassium in a normal range.

Some patients continue to have elevated potassium levels even after using the methods we discussed to prevent and treat elevated potassium. This scenario can justify an early start of dialysis.

### How to Continue ACE/ARB Drugs with Hyperkalemia

The ACE and ARB drugs can raise your potassium and cause a short-term decrease in eGFR. On the other hand, these drugs can slow the long-term loss of your kidney function. These drugs can also be important in the treatment of a weak heart—congestive heart failure. Some kidney and heart specialists will consider a potassium binder drug as a way for their patients to continue ACE or ARB therapy. This is tricky. I recommend that you work with your kidney treatment team and your heart docs to decide whether this approach is right for you.

*Low Potassium—Hypokalemia*

Although not as serious as hyperkalemia, low potassium can also cause problems for patients with CKD. A potassium level below 3.5 is called hypokalemia and can cause nausea and a decrease in your appetite. Low levels of potassium can also cause muscle weakness and heart rhythm problems. At very low levels of potassium, some patients can even experience temporary paralysis.

As your CKD advances, most of you will be on diuretics for blood pressure control, fluid retention, or heart failure. Low potassium is common, especially with high-dose diuretic therapy. Potassium chloride pills or one of the potassium-sparing diuretics can be used to prevent or treat diuretic-related low potassium.

Your kidney team should check your serum potassium within a few weeks of any change in diuretic therapy to look for low potassium. Potassium tablets (potassium chloride) can be taken to treat low potassium and to prevent the diuretic-related low potassium and metabolic alkalosis.

*Diuretics*

There are three main type of diuretics: thiazide diuretics, loop diuretics, and potassium-sparing diuretics (discussed above). The thiazide diuretics include hydrochloro-thiazide (HydroDiuril), chlorthalidone (Diuril), metolazone (Zaroxolyn) and indapamide (Lozol). The loop diuretics include furosemide (Lasix) ethacrynic acid (Edecrin) and bumetanide (Bumex).

Many patients with advanced CKD with or without heart failure may not be getting appropriate diuretic therapy. With advanced CKD, progressively higher doses of loop diuretics may be necessary to get rid of excess body water. Another strategy for resistant fluid accumulation is to combine a loop diuretic and a thiazide diuretic. If you have CKD stage 4 or 5 and a weak heart, taking a thiazide diuretic together with a loop diuretic may help delay the start of dialysis. This combination may also be necessary for patients who have very large amounts of protein in their urine and retain a lot of water.

Some of my patients who had these problems presented with massive swelling of their legs, and sometimes even in their back and abdomen. I had them follow their weight daily at home and saw them at least once a week and sometimes twice a week in my clinic. Many of these patients were able to get rid of the massive amounts of extra fluid and keep the fluid off with the use of these combination diuretics. Use of combination diuretic therapy and close clinical follow-up has helped me to delay the start of dialysis for many of my patients.

But this aggressive diuretic management comes with challenges. One challenge is how to handle the rise in serum creatinine and the fall in eGFR that can occur after large amounts of body fluid are excreted. Part of the rise in serum creatinine may relate to a contraction of blood volume as you get rid of this excess fluid because the creatinine gets more concentrated. But I have been willing to delay dialysis for many such patients, while some of my colleagues have insisted on early start of dialysis in these situations. There is no easy solution. My advice is to discuss your management options with your kidney treatment team. If the fluid keeps coming back, making it hard to breathe and requiring hospitalizations, it may be safer to just "bite the bullet" and start dialysis.

## Patient Example

### *Treatment of Heart Failure Patient with Advanced CKD Without Dialysis*

Here is an example of one of my patients with heart and kidney failure who I managed without dialysis for several years. Mr. B presented with a weight gain of thirty pounds. I used a combination of diuretics to remove the excess fluid. His eGFR went from 20 to 10 after the fluid was removed. I saw Mr. B every week in clinic to manage his heart and kidney problems. Once it became apparent that his kidney function was stable, I saw him every few months for two years, during which he remained off dialysis.

### SUMMARY

The main electrolyte of concern with advanced CKD is potassium. Hyperkalemia, potassium over 6, can result in life-threatening situations. Most hyperkalemia problems can be prevented and easily managed. Patients with advanced CKD need to be aware of the high levels of potassium in Lite Salt and other salt substitutes. Many medications can also raise potassium levels. These include ACE and ARB drugs, potassium-sparing diuretics, and NSAIDs. Diuretic therapy can help decrease hyperkalemia. A low-potassium diet and cooking methods to decrease potassium in foods can also help. Potassium binder drugs may be necessary to control potassium levels and may allow for the continuation of ACE or ARB therapy. Resistant hyperkalemia is an indication to start dialysis.

Metabolic acidosis is another advanced CKD problem. Treatment of metabolic acidosis with sodium bicarbonate may help decrease serum potassium, decrease muscle wasting and atherosclerosis, and may also slow the loss of your kidney function. Diuretic therapy can cause low potassium—hypokalemia—which can be treated with potassium chloride. Combination diuretic therapy can help delay the start of dialysis for some patients with advanced CKD and heart failure. In some cases of advanced CKD and a weak heart, failure of diuretic therapy may lead to an early start of dialysis.

# Chapter 8

## Treatment of the Anemia and Bone Disease Associated with Advanced CKD

TWO OF THE SIGNIFICANT problems that are associated with advanced CKD are anemia and bone and mineral disease (CKD-MBD).

You will learn how to best diagnose and treat CKD-related anemia and iron-deficiency anemia. Both types are common with advanced CKD.

Many treatments for bone and mineral disease are no longer recommended. We will review currently recommended treatments.

### Anemia

Anemia is a condition where your red blood cells are fewer than normal. Anemia can also occur when the red blood cells do not have enough hemoglobin. Hemoglobin is the protein in red blood cells that transports oxygen. The hemoglobin in the red blood cells supplies the oxygen that all of the organs in your body need to function. Without this oxygen these organs cannot function properly.

## Erythropoietin

How anemia connects to CKD is that the kidneys produce a hormone called erythropoietin (EPO). EPO stimulates your bone marrow to make new red blood cells. Bone marrow is the tissue inside the bones of your ribs, back, chest, and pelvis. As kidney function declines, your kidneys make less EPO. This leads to the anemia from CKD.

If you have an eGFR below 30, and even below 60, you may have CKD-related anemia. Luckily, there is a synthetic form of erythropoietin (EPO) that you can take by injection. The manufacture of EPO has dramatically improved life for millions of patients with CKD. I remember the pre-EPO days when CKD patients would have to live with severe anemia. I had patients with hemoglobin levels in the 5 to 6 range, with normal being 14 to 15, and the only option was to be transfused. Repeated blood transfusions, every few weeks or months, were associated with many problems. including fevers, allergic reactions, and production of antibodies that can interfere with kidney transplantation.

### *Other Causes of Anemia in CKD Patients*

One of the most common causes of anemia in CKD patients is an inadequate amount of iron to make red blood cells. Other ingredients the bone marrow needs to make red blood cells are folic acid and vitamin B12. Rarely, a deficiency of these ingredients can cause anemia. Other causes of anemia in CKD patients include blood loss from the GI tract, chronic infections, and other chronic inflammatory states.

### Diagnosing Anemia of CKD

To make a diagnosis of anemia, your health care provider will order a complete blood count, or CBC. This test measures the type and number of blood cells in the body. A diagnosis of anemia is made in males older than age fifteen when their hemoglobin falls below 13 and in females older than age fifteen when their hemoglobin falls below 12. If you have an eGFR below 60 and hemoglobin below the normal level, the cause is likely a decrease in EPO production. Hemoglobin levels gradually decrease as eGFR declines.

Three other blood tests are needed to diagnose anemia of CKD. The first test is a measure of iron levels. The second is the iron-binding protein level. The third is ferritin. The iron level divided by the iron-binding protein level is called the transferrin saturation. The ferritin level measures the amount of iron stored in the body. A transferrin saturation score below 30 percent and/or a ferritin below 200 may mean that in addition to the anemia of CKD, you have iron-deficiency anemia. If you have iron-deficiency anemia, your health care provider may order other tests to look for the source of blood loss, like a colonoscopy to look for polyps or tumors of the colon and an upper endoscopy to look for an ulcer in the stomach.

### What Are the Signs and Symptoms of Anemia in Someone with CKD?

The signs and symptoms may include weakness, feeling tired, headaches, problems with concentration, paleness, dizziness, shortness of breath, and chest pain.

Anemia can also cause problems for your heart. These problems may include an irregular heartbeat or an unusually fast heartbeat. Anemia can also weaken the heart. It can worsen congestive heart failure.

### What Are the Treatments for Anemia Associated with CKD?

### Iron

The first step in treating your anemia is to get iron levels back to normal. Iron pills can get iron levels to a normal range. There are many different types of iron pills: ferrous sulfate, ferrous fumarate, and ferrous gluconate. Look at the dose of any of these iron products that you take. You should get at least 200 mg of iron per day. Generally, you should take around 100 mg of iron twice a day. There are some formulations that can be taken once a day. In order to prevent an upset stomach, you might want to take the iron with food. Do not take your iron with milk, antacids, or calcium pills, because any of these can decrease the amount of iron that is absorbed from your gut. A glass of orange juice can increase the iron absorption. In addition to an upset stomach, some patients experience constipation or heartburn when they take iron pills. If you cannot tolerate iron pills, you can ask your doctor about the possibility of getting the iron you need through your veins, intravenously.

Although folic acid and vitamin B12 deficiency are rare, some kidney doctors routinely give a single pill of these vitamins daily.

### Treating Low Erythropoietin

Today, anemia of CKD can be easily treated with EPO shots, given subcutaneously (under the skin). After many years of EPO use, it was discovered that too much of a good thing can actually be bad for you. When your hemoglobin gets too high, this can increase your blood pressure and your risk of a heart attack or a stroke. EPO therapy is recommended when your hemoglobin is between 9 and 10, with a goal of keeping the hemoglobin below 11.5 to avoid the problems associated with higher hemoglobin levels. In cancer patients, EPO has been shown to increase tumor growth in some cases.

EPO has not eliminated the need for a blood transfusion. If you have a bleeding episode with a big drop in your hemoglobin, you may need a red blood cell transfusion. Transfusions may also be required in situations when you need to get your hemoglobin levels up quickly.

### CKD-Related Bone Disease

Certain minerals and vitamins and a specific hormone are important to keep bones healthy and strong. These minerals are calcium and phosphorus, and the vitamin is vitamin D. The hormone is parathyroid hormone.

As you lose kidney function, you lose the ability to make

the active form of vitamin D. This active vitamin D is made in the kidneys. With a decrease in eGFR, the excretion of blood phosphorus by the kidneys also goes down. High levels of blood phosphorus can cause lower levels of blood calcium. High levels of blood phosphorus, low levels of active vitamin D, and low levels of calcium can work to stimulate the parathyroid glands to release parathyroid hormone into the blood. Parathyroid hormone is produced by the parathyroid glands, which are four pea-size glands in the neck. Parathyroid hormones help raise blood calcium by moving calcium from inside the bones into the blood. The hormone also gets the kidneys to work harder to get rid of more phosphorus. High levels of parathyroid hormone can also cause removal of calcium from bones, which can decrease the strength of your bones.

With progressive CKD, when blood levels of all of these get out of balance, your bones, your heart, and your blood vessels can be affected. The term used by your kidney treatment team to describe this is chronic kidney disease mineral and bone disorder, or CKD-MBD. CKD-MBD can cause bone and joint pain, weak and thin bones, bone fractures, itchy skin, and worsening of anemia. The high blood calcium and phosphorus levels that can come with CKD-MBD can lead to calcification of small blood vessels. Calcified blood vessels can result in infections that won't heal, which can result in amputations, and decreased blood flow to the heart, which can result in heart attacks. The blood vessel complications of CKD-MBD may take many years to appear. To manage CKD-MBD, your blood tests for calcium, phosphorus, parathyroid hormone (PTH), and vitamin D will be monitored.

## Change in Approach to CKD-MBD Treatment

Before I go into the usual approaches to CKD-MBD treatment, I need to explain some of the controversies. KDIGO no longer suggests that we shoot for a normal blood phosphorus level. This change of approach is based on a few factors. Despite all of the treatments we have used for CKD-MBD, which included treatments to get a normal blood phosphorus, there is little evidence that these treatments provided the benefits we hoped for. Elevated phosphorus levels may actually reflect better overall nutrition and may not be all bad.

In the past, kidney specialists like me used a lot of calcium -based phosphorus binders to lower serum phosphorus. I prescribed lots of calcium carbonate (Tums) and calcium acetate (Phoslo) as phosphate binders. This is no longer a recommended therapy because it's been found that these calcium-containing phosphorus binders may lead to calcification of the arteries of the heart and other blood vessels. Many of my patients also received vitamin D type drugs, including the activated vitamin D (calcitriol), which is made in the kidneys. It is no longer recommended to routinely prescribe these calcium binders and vitamin D drugs. Although not proven to be caused by these drugs,, if arterial calcification does occur  it can lead to serious harm.

## Treatment Approaches for CKD-Related Mineral and Bone Disorder (CKD-MBD)

As you will learn in this section the treatments for CKD-MBD have moved away from aggressive use of phosphorus binders and vitamin D analogues.

### *Dietary Phosphorus and CKD-MBD*

One of the most difficult treatment issues for patients with advanced CKD is elevated phosphorus. Phosphorus levels will get progressively higher as kidney function declines. There are basically two ways to decrease phosphorus: (1) a low-phosphorus diet and (2) drugs that bind phosphorus in the gut. Binders are very unpleasant to take. They are called "horse pills" by my patients, since they are so large. To have any benefit, these large pills must be taken with meals.

Another approach to consider is my Smart Diet for CKD. The Smart Diet for CKD is low in phosphorus. As you will recall from chapter 3, this diet can help decrease your risk of atherosclerosis complications and eGFR declines and does help prevent the worsening of CKD-MBD.

Most foods contain phosphorus; however, processed and packaged foods contain especially high levels of phosphorus. Food producers use phosphorus as an additive to preserve the food on the shelf. Try to avoid packaged foods containing ingredients that include the letters "PHOS." The FoodSwitch smartphone app can help you choose the best foods. By avoiding processed foods, you not only decrease your phosphorus intake, but you also decrease your salt and sugar intake, since processed foods are often high in both. Some of the processed foods to avoid are deli meats, hot dogs, crackers, premade meals (including frozen pizza and microwaveable dinners), cheese spreads, and chips.

I will discuss in the last chapter that if you have elevated potassium with an elevated blood phosphorus, the Smart Diet for CKD may not be appropriate, since it tends to be high in potassium.

### *How to Treat Rising Phosphorus and PTH Levels*

If your phosphorus levels get very high and a decrease in diet phosphorus will not bring the levels down, phosphate binders may be considered. The calcium-containing binders may be appropriate if your blood calcium is low.

If your PTH level is high and rising, the first thing to do is try to decrease your blood phosphorus level with the diet adjustments found in chapter 3. If PTH remains high or is increasing, there are three types of drugs that you might receive. These drugs are calcitriol and other vitamin D drugs, and calcimimetics. Some of the vitamin D drugs that can decrease PTH include calcitriol (Rocaltrol), doxercalciferol (Hectorol), and paricalcitol (Zemplar). Cinacalcet hydrochloride (Sensipar) is a calcimimetic that lowers PTH levels by imitating calcium's effects on the parathyroid glands. Cinacalcet is generally reserved for patients who are on dialysis.

If parathyroid hormone levels remain very high after

these treatments, it may become necessary to remove your parathyroid glands surgically. This surgical procedure, which is rarely required, is called parathyroidectomy.

### CKD-MBD and Your Bones

Patients with an eGFR below 60 have increased fracture rates compared with the general population. Some of these fractures may be due to osteoporosis. Osteoporosis is a condition where there is decreased calcium in your bones. Treatment of this disorder in patients with an eGFR below 30 is quite complicated. The drugs that are commonly used to treat osteoporosis can have bad side effects for some CKD patients. Vitamin D may be safe to use for most CKD patients with osteoporosis. Exercising using weights (weight machines, free weights, body-weight exercises) may be helpful to decrease your risk of fractures from thin bones. As you recall, exercise can also decrease your atherosclerosis risk.

Dialysis will not help to control phosphorus or PTH levels. Elevated phosphorus or CKD-related bone disease is not a reason to start dialysis early.

### Acidosis and CKD-MBD

As discussed in chapter 6, approximately half of all patients with an eGFR below 30 will have metabolic acidosis—a bicarbonate of less than 22. Metabolic acidosis can accelerate the loss of bone mineral that comes with CKD-MBD and osteoporosis. Prevention of metabolic acidosis with the Smart Diet for CKD and the treatment of metabolic acidosis with sodium bicarbonate may decrease CKD-MBD and osteoporosis and it may also help slow the decline of your kidney function.

## SUMMARY

One of the biggest problems in the past for patients with advanced CKD was anemia. The anemia of kidney disease is primarily due to low levels of the kidney hormone called erythropoietin (EPO). This hormone, which stimulates the production of red blood cells, is now man-made and readily available. The body's red blood cell factory—the bone marrow—needs building blocks to make red blood cells. These include EPO, iron, B12, and folate. Too high a hemoglobin is not good. Your kidney treatment team will shoot to get your hemoglobin between 10 and12.

The bone and mineral disorder of CKD, CKD-MBD, can lead to fractures, heart attacks, and calcification of your arteries. A decrease in dietary phosphorus as part of the Smart Diet for CKD can not only help decrease serum phosphorus, but it can also help correct metabolic acidosis, which can worsen CKD-MBD. The calcium-containing binders are no longer recommended to lower phosphorus, since they can worsen the calcification of your blood vessels. PTH is elevated in patients with advanced CKD. Mild elevations are okay. If parathyroid hormone levels are very high and rising, your doctor may prescribe calcitriol or other types of vitamin D and calcimimetic drugs to lower your PTH. If these drugs do not work, in rare cases, parathyroid glands may need to be surgically removed.

Dialysis does not improve anemia of advanced CKD; nor

does it help the bone disease of advanced CKD. These problems are not a reason to start dialysis early.

# PART 3

# PREPARING FOR RENAL REPLACEMENT THERAPY

YOUR KIDNEY TREATMENT TEAM may have already brought up the possibility that you will need some form of renal replacement therapy—either dialysis or a kidney transplant). In this section of the book, I will explain why and how you should discuss the possibility of a later start of dialysis with your treatment team. Although most patients with advanced CKD are directed to dialysis, this may not be your best option. The option that is not discussed or promoted enough is a kidney transplant. The best transplant option is to have the transplant surgery before you start dialysis. If this cannot be arranged, a form of home dialysis should be considered as the next best option.

# Chapter 9

## The Timing of Dialysis-- at a Lower eGFR May be the Preferred Approach

THE MAIN GOAL OF this chapter is to help you understand why starting dialysis early, while you have relatively high levels of your own kidney function, is often not beneficial and may in some cases be harmful. First, we'll explore the history of the international trend to start dialysis at higher and higher levels of kidney function. Next, we'll look at the research that supports the start of dialysis at lower levels of eGFR. Since this research depends on eGFR values, we explore the reliability of eGFR to reflect true kidney function.

Like most patients, you may find it hard to understand how starting dialysis early could be a bad idea. The simple answer is that dialysis itself may be harmful. I'll review the potential harms of dialysis.

In general, there are two situations that precede the need for dialysis. One is a planned start of dialysis after a gradual decline of eGFR over many years. The second is when your eGFR drops quickly and unexpectedly and you have an unplanned start of dialysis. Close follow-up by the kidney treatment team is necessary to delay dialysis and to avoid an emergency start of dialysis.

I end the chapter with my recommendations for when you should consider lifelong dialysis.

## A Brief History of the Move to an Earlier Start of Dialysis

In 1979, when I started my forty-year career as a kidney specialist, there were very few dialysis units in South Carolina, where I practice medicine. Dialysis was mostly available for younger, healthier patients. So-called death committees had to decide on who would get the scarce resources of dialysis and transplant. After Medicare began paying for dialysis, for-profit dialysis units sprang up all over the United States. By the 1990s, it seemed that every neighborhood in South Carolina had a dialysis unit. With Medicare coverage of dialysis and transplant and the proliferation of dialysis facilities and transplant programs, many more older and sicker patients were offered these therapies.

Around the year 2000, the notion was promoted that if you started dialysis at higher levels of kidney function, you would live longer. In 1996, one out of three US dialysis patients started dialysis at an eGFR of less than 5. By 2008, only one in ten patients started dialysis at an eGFR of less than 5.

The first published kidney specialist guidelines for when to start dialysis originated in the United States in 1997. These guidelines promoted an early start of dialysis at an eGFR of around 10 or higher. Updated 2006 US guidelines considered starting dialysis at an eGFR over 15. Across Europe, the UK, Australia, and New Zealand, similar early-start guidelines were promoted.

I did not agree with the early-start trend. I decided to do my own research to find out if starting dialysis early was beneficial. The story of a patient I'll call Mr. Smith provided my passion to answer this question.

Mr. Smith was a very pleasant eighty-seven-year-old gentleman. He was sent by his private doctor to my VA kidney clinic. I asked Mr. Smith the reason for his visit. He replied that his doctor told him that he needed to start dialysis very soon. I did my usual exam of Mr. Smith. To my surprise, I found that this poor gentleman had had four separate surgeries to his upper and lower arms. One of the surgeries was to connect an artery to a vein, and the others were to place tubes (grafts) in the forearm and upper arm. The goal for all of the surgeries was to get an access point for blood to flow from Mr. Smith through the dialysis machine and back. Although Mr. Smith had advanced CKD (stage 5), he had stable kidney function for years. On further questioning, I found that Mr. Smith did not have any kidney-failure symptoms. He did not have any problems with his potassium, fluid overload, his appetite, or any other kidney-related symptoms. If I were Mr. Smith's kidney doctor, I would not have put him through any of the surgeries on his arms.

Mr. Smith was very surprised, but relieved, to discover that I felt his need for dialysis was not imminent. I told him he could hold off on dialysis until he had symptoms from advanced kidney failure that could not be managed with medical treatments. I initially saw Mr. Smith every two weeks. When it became clear that his renal function was stable, I changed his visits to once a month. Mr. Smith remained asymptomatic from his kidney failure, without dialysis, for over a year. Then he had a stroke, was hospitalized, and started on dialysis.

There are many patients like Mr. Smith who could delay and potentially never require dialysis. Older adults like Mr. Smith commonly have a slow loss of their kidney function. Some older folks have stable kidney function for years. Like Mr. Smith, many older adults are hospitalized for a non-renal issue that may cause a temporary decline in their kidney function. This decline, although potentially reversible, may influence the medical team to start dialysis.

My research, inspired by Mr. Smith, essentially showed that an early start of dialysis is not beneficial and may be harmful. Since the patients who were started on dialysis early were generally older and sicker, our study looked at more than eighty thousand patients who were under age sixty-five and did not have any major medical issues besides kidney failure. We showed that patients who started dialysis at an eGFR of less than 5 had the longest survival. Other research studies that involved more than a million patients showed that early start of dialysis does not provide a survival benefit. All of the studies mathematically corrected for the fact that patients who start dialysis earlier may be sicker than those who start later.

One might think a CKD patient who starts dialysis early would have a survival advantage due to  the fact that they get medical attention, independent of the dialysis treatment, three times a week in the dialysis unit.The medical attention includes checks of  lab work, blood pressure, physical exam, and medications.. If the same patient did not start dialysis they might only receive medical attention in the doctor's office once a month. The fact that the patient who starts dialysis may not survive as long as the patient followed once a month in the doctor's office, indicates that dialysis itself may be harmful.

## Why an Early Start of Dialysis May Not Be Beneficial and May Even Be Harmful

I have given many talks on the potential harm from starting dialysis too early. Many folks wonder how this can be possible. Dialysis can be lifesaving if you have less than 5 percent of your kidney function remaining. On the other hand, the side effects from dialysis can cause harm. These side effects can outweigh the benefits of dialysis if dialysis is started too early. For example, there can be drops in blood pressure during a dialysis session. These drops in blood pressure can lead to a decrease in blood flow to the heart, brain, and other organs of the body. Also, once you start dialysis, you are likely to lose your remaining kidney function. By the end of your first year on dialysis, most patients have lost all of their remaining kidney function. Even small amounts of your own kidney function and urine output have both survival and quality-of-life benefits because your kidney, even with reduced functioning, works better than a machine.. As you lose your remaining kidney function, you will make less urine. When this happens, you will need to have more fluid removed during your dialysis treatments. More fluid removal and electrolyte shifts during dialysis may contribute to the harms of dialysis. Unfortunately, many patients agree to start dialysis without a good idea of what life will be like as a dialysis patient. A lack of a realistic picture may be one of the reasons why many patients discontinue dialysis treatments.

### Is eGFR a Reliable Marker of Your Kidney Function?

The research that links earlier start of dialysis to shorter survival is based on eGFR. One explanation for the harm that can come from early dialysis is the possibility that the eGFR numbers are not accurate—they may be higher than your actual GFR (see chapter 1). Remember, eGFR is what it says—it's just an estimate of your true kidney function. The estimate assumes that you have a normal amount of muscle for your age and no unusual diet. If you lose weight and body muscle, your eGFR may overestimate your true GFR, measured by twenty-four-hour urine creatinine clearance (see chapter 1). This is because body muscle is the main determinant of your measured GFR. If you lose weight or become malnourished, it is a good idea to follow creatinine-clearance-measured GFR when making a dialysis decision (see chapter 1).

Here is my approach to the eGFR issue. Assuming you have not lost weight or body muscle, your eGFR pattern over time should be a pretty good indicator of the change in your kidney function. If kidney function hasn't declined, any new symptom is probably not due to a change in kidney function. If the kidney team feels that your eGFR data is not reliable, at least two twenty-four-hour urines for creatinine clearance (a measured GFR) should be considered before a dialysis decision is made.

## Early Start of Dialysis for AKI or Emergent Situation

It is important to understand that if you delay starting dialysis and your eGFR is in the 5 to 10 range, you will need close follow-up by your kidney treatment team. Your willingness to consistently follow the CKD treatments prescribed by your kidney team should help you avoid an emergency start of dialysis. These monthly to weekly visits may not be possible if you do not have good medical insurance. It is much easier for kidney doctors to manage advanced CKD patients with dialysis than it is to see them as needed in the outpatient clinic. If a patient is on dialysis, they are seen at least three times a week versus outpatient clinic visits that are usually every few weeks. In the for-profit dialysis world, physicians also have a financial incentive to start dialysis early. The physician fees for dialysis patients are generally much higher than the fees a physician receives for outpatient clinic visits.

Even with close outpatient follow-up, some patients may need an emergency start of dialysis due to an AKI (a short-term large drop in kidney function) episode (see chapter 4). Some of these AKI episodes can lead to an early start of dialysis. This early start might occur after you are admitted to the hospital for a non-kidney issue. One of the most common early-start situations occurs with an episode of worsening CHF. A short-term decline in eGFR in a CHF patient may be due to a combination of weakening of the heart and high doses of diuretics used to treat heart failure. In some of these situations, removing fluids through dialysis can be a lifesaving procedure. In any case, you should not refuse dialysis in an acute emergent situation.

Even so, there are three questions to ask your kidney doctor in these situations:

Will the decline in my kidney function reverse?

Would the doctor consider delaying the start of dialysis to see if your kidney function improves?

Has my kidney function improved after I started dialysis?

Recovery of kidney function is rarely considered once dialysis is started. It is important for you to know that in many AKI situations, kidney function can recover and that once dialysis is started, it may be difficult to see this recovery. Although not a routine practice, your doctor can collect blood and urine samples between dialysis treatments to measure your remaining kidney function.

## When Is It Wise to Start Dialysis?

The 1997–2006 guidelines for kidney doctors concerning when to start dialysis generally supported an early start. This was partly based on the false assumption that dialysis can reverse the weight and muscle loss that often comes with advanced CKD. Much of the push for an earlier start of dialysis connected to these nutrition issues. Although your appetite may improve once you start dialysis, your nutritional indicators, like your blood protein levels and your body muscle, may continue to decline.

As a result of my research and the research by many of my colleagues, there has been a shift away from an early start. The most recent guidelines out of Canada suggest delaying dialysis until an eGFR of 6 unless you have clinical symptoms related to your kidney failure. The 2015 US guidelines recommend a trial of non-dialysis therapy to treat any symptoms of advanced CKD before starting dialysis. If this non-dialysis approach fails, starting dialysis probably makes sense.

## Is There a Lower Limit of eGFR When You Must Start Dialysis?

This is a very interesting question for me. I have been watching the change in attitudes about early start of dialysis. One misconception that encouraged early start is that eGFR will decline relentlessly once you get to an eGFR of 30. This is not the case for many patients. Unfortunately, it is hard to teach an old dog new tricks when it comes to doctors' attitudes. I have to say that in my career I felt compelled to start patients at eGFRs above 5. Nevertheless, when I look at the research on early start, there really is no clear lower limit of eGFR when you must start dialysis. This level will differ from patient to patient.

Here is an example of one of my patients: Mr. K was a very cooperative patient who followed all of my treatment advice.

He had a stable eGFR of 6. I saw him regularly in my clinic to monitor his kidney labs and symptoms. He remained off dialysis with stable kidney labs for three years!

I have given many talks about a later start of dialysis to my US colleagues. After several of these talks, nephrologists came up to me with stories of patients who were able to delay the start of dialysis for months or even years.

If we look at patients in Japan and Taiwan, they rarely start dialysis at an eGFR above 5. My colleagues from Taiwan found that even in their population where most patients started dialysis at an eGFR of around 5 or 6, an earlier start meant worse survival. A summary of the papers on an early start of dialysis that were published between 2001 and 2011 found that for every unit of eGFR higher that a patient started dialysis, their risk of death increased by 3 to 4 percent.

## If You Are Diabetic, Should You Start Dialysis Early?

In the early 1970s, diabetics did not do well on dialysis. Since dialysis was a scarce resource and diabetics did poorly, they were often excluded from dialysis. The good news is that this has changed completely. Today, diabetics do just as well on dialysis as do nondiabetics. A large US study found the same survival disadvantage of an early start in diabetics as in nondiabetics. Thus, there is no reason for diabetics to start dialysis early.

## When Does an Early Start of Dialysis Make Sense?

Patients with CKD often have heart failure. This combination can lead to the retention of fluids and AKI (sudden decline in eGFR). The early start of dialysis in some of these situations may be necessary to manage a patient's shortness of breath and fluid overload. An early start may also be justified if your blood potassium is difficult to control, because high potassium can be life threatening. Most patients can control their potassium with a low-potassium diet, high-dose diuretics, and potassium binder medicines. If this fails, starting dialysis makes sense.

Early start may also be reasonable for patients with a poor appetite, weight loss, and vomiting. Your kidney doctor should be sure there are no other medical problems that are causing these symptoms. As I mentioned, dialysis will probably not reverse malnutrition. On the other hand, dialysis should decrease nausea and vomiting and may improve appetite.

## What Other Symptoms Justify Starting Dialysis?

Most kidney specialists agree that symptoms of kidney failure should be the basis for starting dialysis. Let's look at the symptoms that may lead to dialysis.

According to surveys filled out by kidney doctors, most patients start lifelong dialysis with non-life-threatening symptoms. The most common reported symptoms that "justified" dialysis are weakness, decreased appetite, nausea, and sometimes vomiting. But weakness as a reason to start dialysis does not make sense to me. Weakness may actually get worse with dialysis, and many patients complain of feeling "washed out" after their hemodialysis treatments. Severe nausea and vomiting, as we discussed, however, may justify dialysis.

Other less common symptoms associated with advanced CKD and the start of dialysis include sleepiness, confusion, itching, and hiccups. Confusion is a common reason older adults start dialysis. In many cases, the confusion is not due to advanced CKD and may actually get worse with dialysis. Sleepiness can have many non-CKD causes. Itching may be due to CKD bone disease, which unfortunately does not improve with dialysis. Hiccups are rarely a reason to start dialysis. As mentioned, high potassium and fluid accumulation are two common reasons patients start dialysis.

There are non-negotiable situations that require a patient to start dialysis and are more likely to occur at an eGFR of less than 5. These include seizures, pericarditis (fluid around the heart), and CKD-related bleeding. In each of these cases, non-kidney causes should be ruled out, especially if they occur at eGFR levels above 10.

## SUMMARY

The move to start patients on dialysis at higher levels of their own kidney function was well intentioned but, in my opinion, misguided. In recent years, many patients who were started on dialysis had more than 15 percent of their own kidney function remaining. There is a significant body of evidence to support starting dialysis at lower eGFRs, even below 6. Dialysis can be a lifesaving treatment, but there are also potential harms associated with dialysis. A later start of dialysis can mean additional months to years of time free from dialysis. Patients with eGFRs of less than 15 who hope to delay dialysis need close monitoring by their kidney treatment team. This follow-up can decrease the need for an emergency start of dialysis. An unplanned start of dialysis may come from a bout of AKI (a large drop in kidney function).

The decision to start dialysis should be jointly made by you, your family, and your kidney treatment team. My suggestions in this chapter concerning dialysis start should be shared and discussed with your kidney treatment team. These professionals know and understand all of your personal and medical issues. I am not in a position to know when starting dialysis is appropriate for any reader of this book. Your kidney treatment team will know when it is in your best interest to start dialysis.

Chapter 10

---

# Preparing for Renal Replacement Therapy: Kidney Transplantation, Dialysis, and Dialysis Access

YOUR KIDNEY TEAM MAY have told you that it is time to consider renal replacement therapy—dialysis or a kidney transplant. A preemptive kidney transplant before you ever go on dialysis may be the best option, especially for younger patients who have family or friends willing to donate a kidney. If you do not qualify for a kidney transplant (these reason will be discussed), home dialysis should be considered.

In this chapter, we'll discuss the advantages and disadvantages of the various renal replacement options. If you choose hemodialysis, you will need the connection between an artery and a vein, an AV access, to get your blood to flow through the dialysis machine. Appropriate timing of an AV access can save you from unnecessary surgeries.

## Renal Replacement Options

The two renal replacement options are dialysis and transplant. Dialysis is available in most of the developed world. In the United States and other countries, transplant programs are spread out across large geographic areas. The best option for patients who are eligible is to get a kidney transplant from a blood relative—a live related kidney transplant. A kidney from an unrelated donor—a spouse or a friend—may be as good as one from a relative. The main criteria for a match are the blood type and tissue type of you and the donor (see below). If you are fortunate enough to have a living donor, the very best scenario is a preemptive kidney transplant. By preemptive we mean getting the kidney transplant before you ever go on dialysis. A kidney from someone who dies and donates his or her organs—a cadaver kidney transplant—is the next best choice. To get a cadaver kidney, you will be placed on a kidney transplant waiting list. Most patients are on dialysis for several years before a cadaver kidney becomes available.

## Are You Eligible for a Kidney Transplant?

Your kidney treatment team may not have a local transplant program. Without a local kidney transplant program, you may not be offered this option. In this case, you need to be your own advocate. You should ask your kidney treatment team to send you to the transplant program in your region to see if you are eligible for a kidney transplant. You may have to travel to another city for the transplant workup and surgery. This is well worth the effort.

Different transplant programs have different eligibility

requirements. Most programs exclude patients with life-threatening diseases or conditions. These conditions include non-curable cancers and non-curable infections. Other diagnoses that might exclude you from getting a transplant are severe uncorrectable heart disease, marked obesity, and dementia. Most programs will also exclude patients who do not take their medicines as prescribed and do not follow their doctor's orders. If you have an ongoing drug or alcohol abuse problem, or a serious psychiatric disorder, this may also exclude you from getting a transplant. Regarding your age, most transplant centers discourage kidney transplants for patients over seventy unless they have a healthy kidney donor already lined up. Medicare covers kidney transplant costs in the United States, regardless of a patient's age.

### Advantages and Disadvantages of Kidney Transplant Versus Dialysis

Before you make the decision to get the workup and prepare for a kidney transplant, you need to understand the advantages and disadvantages of the kidney transplant option compared with the dialysis option. Your quality of life after a successful transplant is generally much better compared with dialysis. You avoid the massive time commitment of dialysis. You also avoid the problems associated with hemodialysis access. With a successful transplant, you do not have the food and fluid restrictions that you have with dialysis. Most importantly, a successful kidney transplant can, in most cases, markedly increase your life expectancy compared to dialysis.

On the downside, kidney transplantation is a major surgical procedure that has risks both during and after the surgery. The risks of transplant surgery include infection, bleeding, and damage to the surrounding organs. Although kidney transplant surgery has risks, almost all patients go through transplant surgery without major complications.

Kidney transplant surgery involves placing the transplant kidney in your lower belly. The kidney will be put into the right or left side of your belly, just above the front of your hip bone. The blood vessels of the new kidney are connected to your own blood vessels. The ureter of the transplant kidney (see chapter 1) is connected to your bladder. The operation usually takes about three to five hours. Your transplanted kidney now does the work of two failed kidneys. In almost all cases, you get to keep your own kidneys and the old kidneys stay in your body. After the surgery, you can plan on spending three to four days in the hospital to recover, and it may be a couple of weeks before you can return to work.

There are long-term risks associated with transplantation. You will be required to take several medications daily to decrease the likelihood that your body will reject the transplanted kidney. These anti-rejection medicines decrease your ability to fight infections and cancers, especially skin cancers. Regular health checks by the kidney team can decrease these risks. Sunscreen and regular skin doctor visits can help decrease the skin cancer risk. If you take your transplant medications as directed and get your labs checked frequently, your transplanted kidney can last many years and even decades. The average transplanted kidney lasts around fifteen to twenty years. If your body rejects the kidney, though, you will have to go on dialysis. If this happens, most patients are eligible for and choose to have a second kidney transplant.

### *Your Workup Before You Can Get a Kidney Transplant*

If you meet the eligibility criteria to get a kidney, the next hurdle is the medical evaluation to see if you are healthy enough to get a transplant. The workup should be started early, when your eGFR is around 20 or so. Younger patients should start looking into the transplant option at an eGFR of around 30. The pretransplant workup checks your heart and lung function and does preventive care like a colonoscopy, mammography, and PAP smears for women. In some cases, the workup can take months to complete. You will not be listed on the kidney transplant waiting list or be eligible to receive a living donor transplant until the entire evaluation is completed. Once you are cleared, you are eligible to receive a live donor transplant and the surgery can be scheduled, or you go on the cadaver transplant waiting list.

### *How to Line Up a Kidney Donor*

In order to find out if you have eligible kidney donors, here is my approach. I suggest that you have all family members—parents, children, brothers, or sisters, and any nonrelated potential donors who might be interested—go for a blood draw at the transplant center. Live unrelated kidney transplants have almost the same success rate as a transplant from a relative. Potential nonrelated donors could include good friends, your spouse, or even one of your in-laws. In rare cases, you may even get a kidney from a stranger.

A potential donor has to have a compatible blood type. A donor with blood type O can donate a kidney to patients with any blood type; blood type A can donate to a patient with blood type A and AB; a donor with blood type B can donate to a patient with blood type B and AB, and a donor with blood type AB can only donate to a patient with AB blood. In addition to matching by blood type, there are additional tests used for tissue matching. Tissue matching is made by certain markers on blood cells that are inherited. No one has to know the results of this blood and tissue matching except for the person who has their blood taken. The transplant program can contact the best matches among the potential donors. There is no pressure to say yes to the kidney donation surgery, and this process stays in confidence.

To qualify, potential kidney donors must have normal kidney function and be at least eighteen years old. Things that exclude a donor are being markedly obese, having uncontrolled high blood pressure, diabetes, cancer, HIV, hepatitis, acute infections, and serious mental health conditions. The transplant can take place at a time that is convenient for both you and the donor.

If a potential donor has an incompatible blood type, they may qualify for a paired donor exchange program. The National Kidney Registry will locate a patient who can receive this kidney and find you a kidney that will match.

A disadvantage of living donation is that a healthy person must undergo surgery to remove a healthy kidney. The donor will need some recovery time before returning to work and their usual activities. Changes in surgical techniques have revolutionized kidney donation. Most transplant centers offer robotic, minimally invasive surgery. With this technique, kidney donors have shorter hospital stays (around two days) and recovery time (around two to four weeks). Most living donors get a great deal of satisfaction from their sacrifice. The costs of the donor evaluation and surgery are covered in the United States by Medicare or by your health insurance. There are some expenses that are not covered, however. These include time off from work, travel, and lodging expenses to the transplant center, and incidental expenses. The National Living Donor Assistance Program (www.livingdonorassistance.org) can help with these expenses.

The issue of kidney donor risk needs to be discussed openly. There may be a greater risk of having a future kidney problem for a donor younger than forty-five versus older kidney donors. Some rare issues to consider are what happens if you were to have a trauma to the remaining kidney (as in a car accident) or a tumor in the remaining kidney.

### Preemptive Kidney Transplant Issues

If you are lucky enough to have a living donor, there are some clear advantages to a preemptive transplant. First, you avoid going on dialysis as long as the kidney transplant continues to function. A living donor kidney usually functions immediately. (Some cadaver donor kidneys do not start working for several days. As a result, you may require dialysis until the kidney starts to function.) The whole process of live donor transplant is amazing. I have watched the changes in my patients who received a living donor transplant. They appear to become a new person immediately after the surgery. If you get a preemptive transplant, you can avoid the problems associated with dialysis access. With a preemptive transplant, you also avoid the high first-ninety-days mortality that new dialysis patients face. It turns out that transplant patients' survival may be the highest for those patients who did not have time on dialysis before receiving the kidney transplant.

The trend in the timing of preemptive kidney transplant has mirrored the timing of dialysis. About a third of these transplants occurred at an eGFR above 15 in 2009. In 1995, less than 10 percent of patients who got preemptive transplants had an eGFR above 15. As we discussed in chapter 5, a later start of dialysis may improve your survival. There is no evidence that a later preemptive transplant increases your survival. In my view, an early preemptive transplant is a waste of your own kidney function. More importantly, getting a kidney transplant too early will subject you to more time on drugs that suppress your immune system. This can theoretically increase your chance of a cancer associated with long-term use of these drugs. There also may be a limit to the survival of a transplanted kidney. Getting it too early can theoretically decrease its useful life. Optimally, a preemptive transplant should be scheduled shortly or a few months before you definitely need to initiate dialysis. In order to be able to arrange this, you must complete the pretransplantation workup for both you and your kidney donor well in advance of the planned transplant surgery.

### Cadaver Donor Transplant If No Living Donor Is Available

Assuming that you do not have a live donor, there is a harsh reality that you may have to wait three to five years, or even longer, to get a cadaver transplant. The demand for kidney transplants is far greater than the supply. Blood type O has the longest wait time. If you are blood type O, you can only receive a kidney from a donor with blood type O. Patients with blood type B also have long wait times. If you have had many pregnancies or blood transfusions, you may have a substance in your blood that makes it difficult to match with a cadaver donor.

There are expenses related to cadaver transplant as well. This should be discussed with your kidney treatment team. There are other resources to help with this. Contact NKF Peers Lending Support Program to be matched with a peer mentor who has been in a similar situation. Call 855.NKF.PEERS (855.653.7337) or email nkfpeers@kidney.org.

Here is a very important tip for anyone who wants to decrease the long wait times to get a cadaver donor kidney transplant. It turns out that in order to go on the cadaver donor waiting list, you need to have an eGFR of less than 20. If you go on the waiting list at this early stage of your CKD, you start accumulating wait time. A longer wait time puts you higher on the cadaver transplant recipient list.

I do not recommend that you agree to a cadaver transplant before you have an indication to start dialysis. Nevertheless, it makes sense to discuss the possibility of getting on the waiting list with your kidney treatment team. Ask the team what is needed to get on the cadaver kidney waiting list at your local transplant processing center.

## Dialysis Options

The two types of dialysis are hemodialysis and peritoneal dialysis. For each type of dialysis, you can choose to do the treatment at home or in a dialysis unit. Most kidney doctors would choose home dialysis for themselves. Peritoneal dialysis is almost always performed at home. There is probably no difference in how long you will live if you choose hemodialysis or peritoneal dialysis. Nevertheless, there are advantages and disadvantages of each modality. If you start on one mode of treatment, it is possible to switch to another type as circumstances and your preferences change.

### Peritoneal Dialysis (PD)

Peritoneal dialysis (PD) is a simple form of renal replacement therapy compared to hemodialysis. I encourage you to ask about home PD. There is a push in the United States to get more patients on home PD with more financial incentives to the kidney team. In the past, this form of treatment was not promoted since many facilities did not have experience with PD. You may have to travel to a neighboring treatment facility to get PD training.

*The Home PD Process*

The access for peritoneal dialysis requires a simple surgery. The surgery places a peritoneal dialysis tube in your belly. It is generally recommended to have the catheter placed at least two weeks before beginning PD. After the catheter is placed, you need to keep the area where the tube comes out of the belly clean. It takes about two weeks for the surgical site to heal and for the catheter to be ready to use. Patients who go on to PD do not have to have an AV access (see discussion below). The peritoneal dialysis tube stays in your belly permanently.

When you start PD, you will empty a kind of salty water, called dialysis solution or dialysate, from a plastic bag through your peritoneal dialysis tube into your belly. While the dialysis fluid is inside your belly, it soaks up wastes and extra fluid from your body. There are many different ways to run the fluid in and out. After you receive the training to do PD, you can do the exchanges by yourself. Your kidney treatment team will find the best fluid-exchange schedule for you. Most patients use a machine to automatically run the fluid into and out of your belly overnight while you sleep. This automated peritoneal dialysis machine is called a cycler. Typically, a patient runs the fluid in and out of their belly three to five times per night. Some patients prefer to do the fluid exchanges by hand during the day. This is called continuous ambulatory peritoneal dialysis (CAPD). Each of the exchanges takes about thirty to forty minutes. Most people who do CAPD need four exchanges per day. The last exchange leaves the fluid in your belly while you sleep. You empty the fluid out in the morning and disconnect your tube from the dialysate bag.

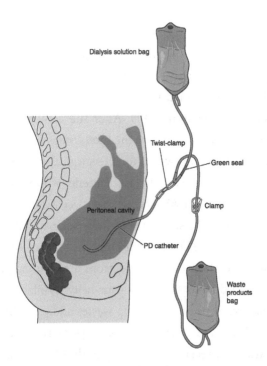

*Dialysis solution bag*

*Twist-clamp*

*Green seal*

*Clamp*

*Peritoneal cavity*

*PD catheter*

*Waste products bag*

### *Advantages of Home Peritoneal Dialysis*

Home peritoneal dialysis is the least complicated type of dialysis that you can do on your own. It does not require the needle sticks of hemodialysis. You can have a flexible schedule that suits you and your lifestyle. You also avoid the travel to and from the dialysis center. You have more time with your family. Since home peritoneal dialysis can be done while you sleep, it doesn't interfere with your normal activities. With nighttime peritoneal dialysis, you can go to work. You can travel with your dialysis fluids and set up treatments anywhere. Because PD is a daily treatment, you won't experience as many ups and downs as you are likely to experience with three-times-a-week hemodialysis. You can also have a more flexible diet and fluid intake compared with the diet restrictions required with three times per week hemodialysis.

### Disadvantages of Peritoneal Dialysis

Not all dialysis centers offer home peritoneal training and support. Although you can do home PD on your own, most patients use family members or friends to help with the PD connections and disconnections. Your PD partner will have to set aside several weeks for training. Sometimes performing PD may stress the relationship between you and you partner. Some patients may not have sufficient space at home to store the peritoneal dialysis cycler machine and PD supplies. Another disadvantage is that PD is done every day, versus three times per week for in-center hemodialysis.

To avoid infections, you must have a clean treatment environment and use good sterile technique when you do your exchanges. Infection in the belly is the biggest problem with PD. You will be taught how to connect and disconnect the peritoneal dialysis tube and fluids using a sterile technique. This will help you avoid infections in the belly, called peritonitis. But the whole process is simple and easy to learn.

## Hemodialysis

In hemodialysis, your blood is pumped through a dialysis machine to remove waste products and excess fluids. You are connected to the dialysis machine using your vascular access (see below). The vascular access allows the dialysis machine to pump your blood through a filter (dialyzer) and then return the filtered blood to your body.

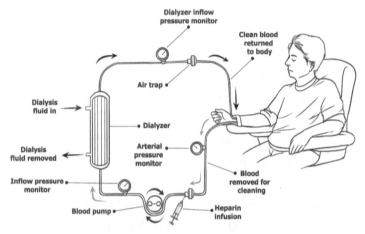

Hemodialysis can be done at a dialysis center or at home. When done in a center, it is most commonly done three times a week and takes between three and five hours per session. Home hemodialysis is generally done three times a week. Some home hemodialysis patients opt for more frequent, shorter treatments at home.

### Advantages of In-center Hemodialysis

Dialysis centers are available in most parts of the developed world. In these centers, you have trained health care providers to be with you at all times during your hemodialysis treatments. Some patients are happier to have a trained dialysis staff member perform their treatment, versus a trained family member or friend who could do the treatment at home. Dialysis in center also eliminates the need to keep dialysis equipment and supplies in your home. Some patients like the social aspect of going to a dialysis facility. In-center hemodialysis is less of a time commitment for the dialysis treatments, compared with daily or nightly home peritoneal dialysis.

### Disadvantages of Hemodialysis

Compared with nightly or daily PD, if you choose three-times-per-week in-center hemodialysis, you have a longer time between treatments. Three hemodialysis treatments per week may mean stricter limits on your diet and the liquids you take in between treatments. If you dialyze only three days a week, you will require faster fluid removal during hemodialysis compared with daily fluid removal by PD. Fast fluid removal during hemodialysis can drop your blood pressure and stress your heart. These low-blood-pressure episodes may be accompanied by light-headedness, shortness of breath, abdominal cramps, nausea, or vomiting. Remember when I tried to explain how early start of hemodialysis may be harmful? These blood pressure drops are one of the factors. You may not have symptoms from some of the drops in blood pressure. Nevertheless, these drops can decrease blood flow to vital organs, especially your heart. This can increase your risk of a heart attack and heart failure.

Low blood flow to your brain and kidneys can damage these organs as well. Low blood pressure is much less common with peritoneal dialysis when compared to hemodialysis. During hemodialysis, many patients have muscle cramps and some people feel washed out after treatments. Recovery from this washed-out feeling may take several hours. These ups and downs from the three-times-per-week hemodialysis sessions are much less common with daily PD treatments.

Another disadvantage of hemodialysis is the need for a blood-flow access. You may need multiple access surgeries to get an access that gives adequate blood flow for the hemodialysis machine. Every time you go on hemodialysis, two large needles are placed into this access. The access can get infected and may also clot off. This closure may require another surgery or an x-ray procedure to open it up. Many patients do not have a working access in their arm when they start hemodialysis. In these cases, you may require a catheter placed in a neck vein to remove and return your blood. This central venous catheter (CVC access), often gets infected and may clot off.

Many patients who receive in-center hemodialysis are either unable to work or choose not to work. Hemodialysis treatments usually require travel to and from the dialysis center. If you want to work during the day, in rare cases, nighttime in-center hemodialysis may be available. Some patients are trained to do hemodialysis in their home, and they can do the dialysis at night and work during the daytime, which I will discuss below.

### Incremental Hemodialysis

Some nephrologists suggest so-called incremental hemodialysis when a patient first starts on dialysis. This means that patients start with two instead of three dialysis sessions per week. To opt for this decrease in weekly dialysis time, patients are usually required to have more than 10 percent of their own kidney function. As a patient's own kidney function declines, they are moved to three-times-per-week treatments. Thus, incremental hemodialysis requires early start of dialysis. I personally do not recommend this type of treatment. I suggest that patients delay dialysis until they have an indication to start three-times-a-week conventional hemodialysis.

### Home Hemodialysis

This is a much more difficult technique to learn compared with home PD. Nevertheless, some patients prefer to do three-times-per-week hemodialysis treatments in the evenings at home rather than in a dialysis center. Smaller hemodialysis machines make this treatment easier. All of the equipment to perform home hemodialysis is supplied by the dialysis center. In an effort to make hemodialysis a more continuous treatment, some patients do short treatments (two to three hours), five or six nights per week. Some patients claim that they feel better with five or six weekly treatments compared with three treatments per week. I personally do not feel that the advantages of so-called frequent hemodialysis outweigh the downsides of this approach. One big disadvantage is that more frequent dialysis requires more needle sticks. This can lead to a need for more access surgeries.

## The Challenges of Hemodialysis Access

### AV Fistula

An arteriovenous—AV—fistula is the best hemodialysis access. For an AV fistula surgery, your surgeon connects an artery to a vein in your forearm or in your upper arm. Here is an illustration of what an AV fistula looks like if the surgery is done at the wrist.

To get to your blood vessels, the surgeon

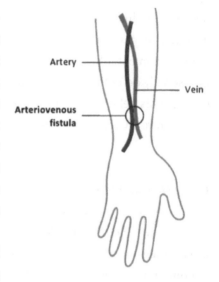

makes a small incision at your wrist level or just above the bend of your elbow. Normally your blood is pumped from your heart into your arteries. Next your blood returns to your heart through your veins. When your surgeon creates an AV fistula, part of the blood that passes out of your artery goes directly into the vein. The blood comes into your veins at a high enough pressure to be pumped through the dialysis machine. The high pressure in the vein makes the vein bigger and thicker. These bigger veins can accommodate the two dialysis needles that are required to get your blood to the dialysis machine and then back to your fistula. After the surgery, it can take six weeks to three months before the hemodialysis staff can use your new fistula.

Finding a vascular access had been called the Achilles' heel of hemodialysis. The first challenge is to find a suitable vein that a surgeon can connect to an artery in one of your arms to form the AV fistula. Most patients who develop end-stage kidney failure have many blood draws and many IVs before they go on dialysis. All of these needle sticks can make the veins in your arms useless for an access.

One thing all advanced CKD patients need to learn is that you must try to preserve the veins in your arms. Several years ago at a kidney meeting on dialysis access, I learned about an interesting way to preserve your veins. One of the speakers had a great slide, which showed a tattoo on the forearm of a CKD patient. The tattoo was of a skull and crossbones and read "no needle sticks in this arm." This is certainly one way to drive home the point. Any CKD patient with an eGFR below 30 should protect the veins in your nondominant arm and not let anyone stick the veins in your left arm if you are right-handed, and no sticks in your right arm if you are left-handed. The reason is simple: If you need to go on hemodialysis, you would like to have the hand you prefer to use available during the treatment. By avoiding needle sticks in your nondominant arm, you can decrease the need for multiple surgeries to get a working dialysis access.

Mapping of your veins before surgery and a highly experienced vascular surgeon can increase the likelihood that the access surgery will be successful. Younger patients and patients with large, prominent veins in their forearms may get a working dialysis access after one operation. Nevertheless, it is often necessary for patients with few or small veins in their arms to have several operations before they have a well-functioning dialysis access.

Of course, these surgeries can be minimized or eliminated altogether if you get get a preemptive kidney transplant, or by choosing peritoneal dialysis.

### Other Types of AV Access

There are several choices for hemodialysis access. An AV fistula has the longest life and the least number of complications. In some cases, your veins may not be large enough or strong enough to connect to an artery. In some of these cases, the surgeon may place a tube, or graft, in your forearm or upper arm. One advantage of a graft is that it can be used in days to weeks, instead of months.

The last choice for dialysis access is a CVC. The preferable location for insertion of the CVC are the large veins in your neck, the internal jugular veins. In some cases, a catheter can be placed in a vein in your chest—the subclavian vein, or leg—the femoral vein. Of all access choices, a CVC has the most complications. Infections are common and often lead to hospitalizations. In the United States and other countries, the vast majority of patients are started on dialysis with a CVC. Only one in five patients in the United States starts dialysis with an AV fistula. The AV fistula is the preferred access since it rarely clots off or gets infected. Delaying dialysis until you have a working AV access may be another reason for a later start of dialysis.

**Timing of Hemodialysis Access**

Another challenge regarding AV access is when to undergo surgery. I encourage you to use the prediction tools from chapter 6, to see if you will need dialysis in the future. If your CKD 3 (eGFR 30–60) remains stable, you do not have to worry about dialysis access. If you have an eGFR of less than 30, access surgery should be discussed with your kidney team. My approach is to individualize the decision. If you are a younger patient (for dialysis patients that is around sixty or younger), I generally suggest putting in a dialysis access sooner rather than later. The reason for this advice is that younger patients generally have better veins compared with older patients and are more likely to need dialysis. Also, a working fistula can get better with time and can help you avoid a CVC.

I am much more inclined to delay access surgery for my older patients. For some older patients, a CVC access may be justified in order to avoid multiple painful access surgeries (see the story of Mr. Smith, chapter 8).

More than half of newly created AV accesses do not work in older adults. Often patients with a failed access go through multiple radiologic or surgical interventions to try to get the access to work. If you are an older patient who has agreed to dialysis, your access should not be placed more than six months before dialysis is expected to start. In some cases a graft (tube in your arm) may be preferred, since it can be used after a few weeks

## Patient Example

*Preparing for renal replacement therapy.*

Here is an example of one of my patients who went through the process of preparation for renal replacement therapy. Mr. H is a sixty-year-old diabetic patient who had a good bit of urine protein and an eGFR of 15 when I first saw him. Over the next year, his eGFR declined to the 6 to 8 range. He was very resistant to the idea of dialysis and the surgery for a vascular access. He was hoping to get a preemptive transplant from a family member or friend. The one potential donor, a friend, decided against the transplant surgery. He had the veins in his arms mapped for a possible fistula, but his veins were quite small. After talking to a patient who was on home PD, he and his wife agreed that peritoneal dialysis would be their best bet. Mr. H had a peritoneal catheter placed in his belly and he and his wife went through the PD training. He is on the cadaver transplant waiting list and is doing well on nightly home PD.

### SUMMARY

If you have an eGFR of less than 30, or if you are losing your kidney function quickly, it is time to prepare for renal replacement therapy. The best option, especially for younger patients, is to get a preemptive kidney transplant before ever going on dialysis. You need to ask your kidney team about this option. Start early in your search to recruit potential kidney donors. You might be surprised to learn that some of your family members, your spouse, or even your friends would consider donating one of their kidneys. There does not appear to be any benefit to receiving a kidney transplant early, at an eGFR over 10. If you do not have a donor, be sure to get on the waiting list to receive a cadaver transplant, possibly at an eGFR of around 20. Early listing can potentially decrease your wait time for a kidney.

Your next best option may be home peritoneal dialysis (PD). If you choose hemodialysis, you will most likely receive your treatments in a dialysis unit. To do hemodialysis you will need an AV access. You may avoid multiple access surgeries by not allowing needle sticks in the vein to be used for access. Access surgeries should be delayed in older adults until you are about six months away from starting dialysis. Assuming that you don't need to start emergently, dialysis should be delayed until you have a working AV access.

# Chapter 11

## Dr. Ro's Pearls of Wisdom

I OFFER THE READER the highlights of each of the ten chapters in the book. Some of you may prefer to start here and then go to each chapter for a more detailed discussion.

### Chapter 1: The Basics of Kidney Anatomy and Function

The measure of your kidney function that I refer to in this book is the estimated glomerular filtration rate, or eGFR.

The eGFR is the lab result your doctor gets from your blood test.

The eGFR is a measure of the rate that blood is filtered through the tiny blood vessels in the kidney, which make up the glomeruli—thus the term "glomerular filtration."

eGFR is based on the level of serum creatinine. Creatinine is a marker used to measure glomerular filtration. There is no reason to try any natural or herbal remedies to lower your serum creatinine. This will not affect your kidney function. These "home" and "natural" remedies can be harmful!

The kidneys are fist-size organs—each kidney connects to a tube, a ureter, and the two ureters connect to the bladder.

Urine is produced from the glomerular filtrate as it flows

through a tube from the glomerulus. It eventually gets to the bladder and passes out the urethra, which is in a man's penis and a woman's vulva area.

The change of your eGFR over time is what really matters.

You may have an eGFR in the 50 range that can move down to 45 or up to 55 without any real change in your kidney function; don't get upset about any single eGFR number. A small change in your eGFR up or down is not important, has no real meaning. You need to look at the longer-term picture of your eGFR pattern over months and years.

Your kidney team should base the management of your CKD on how fast your eGFR is declining. For many patients, eGFR remains the same for years.

Five stages of CKD are used in this book. To avoid confusion, I do not use the newer staging system that adds additional stages and includes urine protein levels.

If you have stage 1 and 2 CKD, an eGFR over 60, it is unlikely that you will have a serious kidney issue unless you also have a large amount of protein in your urine.

Patients with stage 3 CKD, with an eGFR of 30 to 60, rarely face a dialysis decision.

The vast majority of the world's CKD population has stage 1, 2 and 3 CKD.

Stage 4 CKD is an eGFR of 15 to 30; Stage 5 CKD is an eGFR of less than 15.

Stage 5 CKD has been called kidney failure. I disagree with this term since it implies that you need dialysis when your eGFR is less than 15.

To me "kidney failure" is the point where you need dialysis or a kidney transplant. This usually becomes necessary when your eGFR is less than 10 and for some patients less than 5.

Your estimated GFR lab result may not be accurate if you have lost a significant amount of body weight and body muscle.

If there are questions about the accuracy of your eGFR, a twenty-four-hour urine collection for creatinine clearance, a measured GFR—not just an estimated GFR—should be done.

For most patients, following the change of your eGFR over time is a useful way to follow your CKD.

Urine protein levels are the most important predictor of how fast your kidney function will decline.

ACE and ARB drugs, discussed throughout the book, are the most important drugs to decrease urine protein and possibly slow the decline of eGFR.

You can tell if you are getting an ACE if the generic name, not the trade name, of your blood pressure pill ends in "pril" (like captopril).

You can tell if you are getting an ARB if the generic name of your blood pressure drug ends in "tan" (like losartan).

In addition to following your eGFR, it is a good idea to follow your urine protein levels.

A urine dipstick can give an idea of the amount of the protein called albumin in your urine. Another test your doctor may follow is the urine "spot" protein. For this test, a small amount of urine is sent to the lab to estimate how much albumin you pass in your urine in a day.

## Chapter 2: What You Can Do to Lower Your Risk of "Hardening of the Arteries"—Atherosclerosis

For any patient with CKD, one objective for reading this book is to decrease your atherosclerosis risk, which can potentially increase your lifespan by years.

Atherosclerosis is the hardening and the narrowing of your arteries by a waxy substance called plaque that builds up over many years.

The main clinical problems that can happen when atherosclerosis progresses include heart attack, stroke, worsening kidney function, and decreased blood flow to your legs, which can lead to resistant infections and amputations.

Lifestyle changes are strongly encouraged to slow progressive atherosclerosis.

Stop smoking; this may be the most important thing you can do to decrease your chances of a heart attack, stroke, or blood-flow problem to your legs.

A regular exercise schedule may be the "fountain of youth," since it not only can decrease atherosclerosis, but exercise can also improve your overall physical and brain health.

Monitor your blood pressure to avoid too low a blood pressure; less than 90 systolic—top number—can be dangerous.

Try to get eight hours of sleep a night and do things to relax; this will also decrease your atherosclerosis risk.

Most patients with CKD will require cholesterol medications to get their "bad" cholesterol, their LDL, below 100.

Raising the so-called good cholesterol, the HDL, has not been shown to decrease atherosclerosis issues.

Diabetics are at a high risk of severe atherosclerosis and should aim for an LDL below 70.

Despite a lot of research, it is unclear whether high blood sugar levels, by themselves, increase the severity of your atherosclerosis.

To avoid the possible harms of low blood glucose, younger diabetics should shoot for a hemoglobin A1C of 6 to 7, while older diabetics should aim for an A1C of 7.5 to 8.

Daily foot care and annual eye exams can help diabetic CKD patients avoid amputations (from lower extremity infections) and blindness (from diabetic eye diseases).

A decrease in added salt to food may help decrease blood pressure and atherosclerosis risk.

ACE and ARB drugs not only have the potential to decrease urine protein and loss of eGFR, but they may also decrease atherosclerosis risk.

## Chapter 3: The Smart Diet for CKD

Avoid diet supplements. They can make your kidney disease worse. Supplements are not tested by the FDA to see if they are safe and if they have any benefits. They may have impurities, as well as high amounts of potassium and phosphorus.

My Smart Diet for CKD may help decrease obesity, atherosclerosis, blood vessel disease of CKD, diabetes, hypertension, loss of kidney function, buildup of acids from progressive CKD, bowel cancer, and irritable bowel symptoms of alternating constipation and diarrhea.

The Smart Diet for CKD is relatively low in protein, avoids foods with added sugar and high levels of carbohydrates, encourages more whole-grain foods and fewer refined grains, has more fiber and less saturated fat, sodium, and phosphorus.

A high-protein diet may not only be harmful to the kidneys, but it may also worsen the retention of acids that comes with progressive CKD.

The Smart Diet for CKD is a relatively low-protein diet since it provides much of your protein from plant sources, fruits, and vegetables.

A low-protein diet is also generally low in saturated fat, cholesterol, sodium, and phosphorus, while it has lots of fiber.

A true low-protein diet is around 0.3 grams of protein per pound of your weight. The Smart Diet for CKD roughly shoots for this protein intake. There is no reason for patients who have an eGFR over 30 and who are not losing kidney function quickly to go on a very-low-protein diet, which is around 0.16 grams of protein per pound of your body weight per day.

Very-low-protein diets can lead to malnutrition, especially in older adults who may require a higher protein intake. A very-low-protein diet can exacerbate the decline in nutritional status that comes with progressive CKD.

Learn to read food labels to decrease portion size, sugars, saturated fats, unrefined grains, phosphorus, and salt intake while you try to increase diet fiber, whole grains, vegetables, fruits, low-fat dairy, and fish.

Shoot for total daily calories of 10 to 15 per pound of body weight. Calorie intake for weight loss depends on your exercise level, age, height, and current weight—see www.healthline.com.

Weight loss tips: If you do not need to restrict water due to advanced CKD or heart disease, drink water before meals to reduce hunger; more protein and fewer carbs will increase calories you burn; exercise decreases muscle loss with weight loss and helps increase your life span and life quality; cut portion sizes, because our American ones are way too big.

Try to avoid foods with added sugar, honey, and syrupy foods, candy, cakes, ice cream, pastries, sweetened beverages, and especially sodas.

Most of the foods in an average diet contain refined grains that are low in fiber, for example: bagels, corn bread, muffins, bread crumbs, biscuits, crackers, white breads, pretzels, pizza, cakes, cookies, tortillas, waffles, white rice, noodles. These should be avoided.

Saturated fats are found in the greatest amounts in lard, butter, shortening, egg yolks, red meat, whole milk, beef fat, coconut, palm oils, fatty meats, dairy, cakes, cookies, and fast foods like pizza. These, too, should be avoided.

You get more fiber in your diet by leaving the skins on your fruits and vegetables and by choosing whole fruit over fruit juice.

By increasing fiber in your diet, you reduce your diabetes risk, decrease constipation and other irritable bowel symptoms, and decrease your risk of colon cancer.

The Smart Diet for CKD avoids processed meats such as cold cuts, canned foods, frozen foods, prepared meals, organ meats like liver, dairy products that are not fat free, and bottled beverages, especially sodas.

## Chapter 4: Reversible Declines in Kidney Function

Dehydration is the most common reason patients with CKD have a temporary worsening of kidney function. This temporary decline in eGFR is called acute kidney injury, or AKI.

Vomiting, diarrhea, and high fever can all cause dehydration.

A severe form of AKI is called ATN: acute tubular necrosis. This form of AKI may occur after prolonged declines in blood pressure; ATN can require short-term dialysis.

If you start dialysis after an AKI, be sure to ask your doctor if your kidney function has recovered and whether you can come off dialysis.

To avoid an AKI episode, stay well hydrated and drink plenty of fluids. This is especially important if you are sick from a viral illness or flu, or if you are taking a medicine that can cause a decline in your kidney function.

Drugs that can cause a decline in kidney function include ACEs and ARBs, PPIs like Prevacid and Nexium, used for heartburn, NSAIDs used for pain and fever, like Motrin and Advil, and x-ray contrast.

Too much blood pressure medication can also decrease eGFR.

If you have a weak heart, and especially if you are on high-dose water pills (diuretics), your kidneys may behave as if you are dehydrated and your eGFR can go down.

If CHF problems are severe and recurrent, with decreased eGFR and severe shortness of breath, some patients may need to start dialysis.

In men, one of the most common causes of eGFR decline is

blockage of urine flow by a large prostate (BPH, benign prostatic hypertrophy). This AKI is easily treated and usually will reverse after a catheter is passed into the bladder.

## Chapter 5: What You Can Do to Slow the Decline of Your Kidney Function

The five main causes of CKD are diabetes, hypertension, atherosclerosis, glomerular diseases, and polycystic kidney disease (PCKD).

The factors we discuss in this chapter to slow kidney function decline apply to all of these causes of CKD.

Some patients with PCKD may qualify to receive a new drug to slow the decline of kidney function: tolvaptan.

Some diabetics with CKD may benefit from drugs called SGLT2 inhibitors. These drugs help with blood sugar control and may also decrease urine protein and slow the decline of eGFR.

Blood pressure goals for CKD patients depend on your risk of losing kidney function.

Patients with high levels of urine protein are likely to lose kidney function quickly. For these patients, the goal blood pressure is 110–120 over 70–80.

130 over 80 is a goal blood pressure for all other CKD patients.

Too low a blood pressure, below around 90 systolic (top number), can be dangerous. It can worsen kidney function. It may also cause a decreased blood flow to the heart and the brain, which can result in a heart attack or a stroke.

If you are feeling weak or dizzy, take your blood pressure before you take your next dose of medicine. If your blood pressure is 90–100 systolic, suspend taking your next dose of blood pressure medicine. Discuss this approach with your kidney team.

For better blood pressure control, ask your doctor to make your blood pressure dosing once a day and find out if you are on a water pill (diuretic), usually HCTZ, in addition to your other blood pressure meds. Taking blood pressure medications before bed may produce better results than daytime dosing.

If you have more than 1+ protein in your urine, an ACE or an ARB drug (not both) is the key to slowing the loss of your kidney function.

If you have high levels of urine protein, you need to ask your doctor if you can continue the ACE or ARB even if you get an initial drop in eGFR after the ACE or ARB is started. This is a common situation.

The ACE or ARB can decrease urine protein, decrease progressive atherosclerosis, and decrease loss of kidney function.

There is no proven benefit to your kidneys from drinking a lot of water, unless you have kidney stones.

Even though a low-protein diet has not been proven to slow the loss of your kidney function, the Smart Diet for CKD patients tends to also be low in protein as well as saturated fats and is high in fiber and whole grains, which all have general health benefits and may contribute to slowing loss of kidney function.

In addition to the Smart Diet for CKD, you may need sodium bicarbonate pills to correct a low bicarbonate-metabolic acidosis (see chapter 7). This may help slow loss of kidney function and decrease muscle breakdown that comes with low levels of kidney function.

Very-low-protein diets, with keto-acid supplements, in my opinion, are not appropriate for the vast majority of CKD patients. This type of diet may slow loss of kidney function for some CKD patients with an eGFR below 30 who are not diabetic. I would consider this diet for patients with high levels of urine protein, who are more likely to lose kidney function rapidly. To avoid malnutrition, this diet should be supervised by a licensed dietician. The keto-analog supplements can help decrease the risk of malnutrition. This type of diet is very difficult for most patients to follow.

Because of the likelihood of a slow loss of kidney function in older adults and the high likelihood of a decline in your nutritional state, I do not recommend low or very-low-protein diets for older adults with CKD.

## Chapter 6: A Look into the Crystal Ball: How Likely Is It that You Will Need Dialysis in the Future?

There are three ways to predict whether you will need dialysis. Use these methods with your kidney treatment team to find out the likelihood that you will need dialysis.

Your urine protein level is the main determinant of how quickly you will lose kidney function and whether dialysis may become necessary.

One simple way to predict dialysis is to plot your eGFR

data. When you look at these eGFR results, you can calculate the average loss of eGFR in units per year.

The normal rate of eGFR loss is around 1 unit per year. People that wind up on dialysis generally lose kidney function faster than 5 units of eGFR per year.

In general, the older you are, the slower the loss of your kidney function.

Most older patients do not have high levels of urine protein. This may partly explain their slower loss of kidney function as well as the fact that older patients can have a stable eGFR, below 30, for years.

On average, if your eGFR is below 30, around one in three younger patients and one in fifteen older patients wind up needing dialysis.

Delaying dialysis until your eGFR reaches the 5 to 10 range will decrease the likelihood that older patients will need dialysis.

Many older adults with an eGFR of less than 30 will die of another cause before they ever need dialysis.

Sudden drops in eGFR—known as AKI—account for around 10 percent of the people who wind up on dialysis. The need for dialysis after an AKI cannot be predicted. If you start dialysis after an AKI, be sure to ask your kidney doctor to look for recovery of your kidney function. This is not a routine practice.

## Chapter 7: Electrolyte and Diuretic Management in Advanced CKD

Advanced CKD is an eGFR around 30 or less.

High potassium can be life threatening, especially if blood potassium rises quickly. A slow rise in potassium over weeks to months is much less dangerous.

Prevention of high potassium is crucial. If your potassium is elevated, you should avoid Lite Salt (potassium chloride). Also avoid potassium-sparing diuretics: spironolactone, triamterene, amiloride.

ACE and ARB drugs can raise potassium. You should be taking a water pill (like HCTZ) with your ACE or ARB to make them more effective and to avoid high potassium.

If you have high levels of urine protein and you are losing kidney function rapidly, some kidney specialists will continue the ACE or ARB despite a decline in eGFR or a rise in potassium.

ACE and ARB drugs may be especially important to slow loss of kidney function for those patients who are losing kidney function rapidly.

A low-potassium diet, or a medicine that binds the potassium in your diet, may be necessary for you to continue the ACE or ARB. This approach needs to be discussed with your kidney treatment team.

The Smart Diet for CKD is relatively high in potassium and therefore some of the recommended foods will not be appropriate if you have problems with high potassium. Check with your kidney team dietician.

If your potassium cannot be safely managed by avoiding the drugs that raise potassium, use of a low-potassium diet and potassium binders, dialysis is indicated.

Acids build up in the blood with advanced CKD. A

Steven Rosansky

low-protein diet, part of the Smart Diet for CKD, and oral sodium bicarbonate may help correct acidosis.

Correcting the acidosis of CKD may slow the loss of kidney function, decrease the nutritional deterioration of progressive CKD, decrease insulin resistance that can decrease atherosclerosis, and help prevent an elevated potassium.

With progressive CKD, you may have a buildup of fluids in your body—first seen as edema, or swelling in your ankles.

With an eGFR of less than 30, a loop diuretic (Lasix, Bumex, and Edecrin) may work better than the diuretic HCTZ.

A common problem with high-dose diuretics is low potassium and high bicarbonate. Potassium chloride or potassium-sparing diuretics are used to treat this problem—watch out for high potassium.

Patients with a weak heart and CKD may start dialysis early if diuretic and heart failure treatments fail to control fluid buildup and shortness of breath.

## Chapter 8: Treatment of the Anemia and Bone Disease Associated with Advanced CKD

Anemia is a condition where your red blood cells are fewer than normal.

EPO, also called erythropoietin, is made by normal kidneys. As kidney function declines, less EPO is produced. This EPO is now available as an injection.

EPO stimulates the production of red blood cells in the center of long bones called the bone marrow.

176

Hemoglobin is the protein in red blood cells that transports oxygen. All the cells in your body need oxygen to function.

When you are treated for the anemia of CKD, you will have your iron checked. Many patients with anemia of CKD will need iron in addition to EPO to treat their low hemoglobin and low red cell count.

If your EPO dose leads to a hemoglobin level over 12, this can increase your blood pressure and your risk of heart attacks and strokes. Your kidney treatment team will need to adjust your dose of EPO.

CKD-MBD is the abbreviation for the mineral and bone disorder of CKD. It involves vitamin D, the minerals calcium and phosphorus, and the hormone PTH.

The kidneys not only make EPO, but they also make the active form of vitamin D.

Kidneys are key to regulating blood levels of phosphorus. As kidney function declines, your ability to get rid of phosphorus and make active vitamin D also declines.

PTH is involved with keeping the levels of phosphorus and calcium in a normal range through the effects of PTH on the kidneys and your bones.

Elevated levels of calcium and phosphorus can cause your blood vessels to calcify, harden, and worsen atherosclerosis. This can lead to heart attacks and amputations.

The bad effects of calcium and phosphorus on blood vessels are rare. In the past, kidney doctors prescribed very large pills to take with meals to bind phosphorus. Some of these pills contained calcium. The calcium binders may be harmful (may increase calcium in the arteries) and are no longer recommended. There are non-calcium-containing phosphorus binders. These drugs may be necessary if your phosphorus levels get very high.

Abnormal levels of vitamin D, phosphorus, calcium, and PTH can make your bones weak.

I encourage you to decrease the amount of phosphorus you eat. This may not only be good for your blood vessels (decreases hardening of the arteries), but it may also slow the decline of your kidney function and may help your bones stay healthy. Low phosphorus is part of the Smart Diet for CKD patients.

Things that are high in phosphorus include packaged and processed foods (phosphorus is added to give these foods a longer shelf life), red meats, and dairy products. Many of the foods to avoid in the Smart Diet for CKD are often high in phosphorus. These include deli meats, hot dogs, crackers, premade meals, including frozen pizza and microwaveable dinners, cheese spreads, and chips.

If your PTH levels are high, one of the active vitamin D medicines are recommended. Vitamin D is not routinely recommended for CKD patients who do not have high PTH levels. The reason is that vitamin D can increase phosphorus and calcium levels, which can have harmful effects on your blood vessels.

## Chapter 9: The Timing of Dialysis- at a Lower eGFR May be the Preferred Approach

I encourage you to read the story of Mr. Smith. He was

prepared for dialysis far too early.

The reason kidney doctors moved to starting dialysis at higher levels of eGFR was to improve patient survival.

My research and the research of many of my colleagues show just the opposite effect, which is shorter survival with earlier start of dialysis.

It is reasonable to delay dialysis until an eGFR below 10 and for some patients until an eGFR of around 5.

In several studies, patients who started dialysis at an eGFR of 5 or less had the best survival.

There is no reason to start dialysis solely for your eGFR number.

Since dialysis itself can be harmful, to justify starting dialysis, you should have symptoms of kidney failure that cannot be managed without dialysis.

The possible harms of hemodialysis include a decrease in the blood flow to your heart, brain, and other vital organs.

By one year after you start dialysis, it is very likely that you will lose all of your own kidney function. Even at low levels of function, your own kidney function has survival and quality-of-life benefits.

Dialysis may improve your appetite, but it does not improve your overall nutrition. Your nutritional state generally declines with time on dialysis.

Other possible downsides to starting dialysis include more days in the hospital, muscle cramps on the machine, feeling washed out after a dialysis treatment, and a decrease in physical and mental abilities, especially for older patients.

If you are going to safely delay dialysis, you need close follow-up by your kidney team.

AKI (sudden unexpected declines in kidney function) can result in an emergency start of dialysis.

Patients with CHF and CKD may have severe shortness of breath and fluid retention that cannot be managed without dialysis. This combination can lead to an early start of dialysis.

If your potassium level cannot be controlled, you may need to start dialysis.

Poor appetite, vomiting, and weight loss with no other explanation other than your kidney problem is a reason to start dialysis.

Starting this lifelong treatment is a decision that you and your family must make together with your kidney team.

Every patient and situation is unique. The suggestions I provide concerning when to start dialysis are not treatment recommendations. Use this information to discuss your particular situation with your kidney treatment team.

I am not your kidney doctor, and every patient and situation is different. Your kidney treatment team is best qualified to help you make the final decision regarding dialysis and your other kidney treatments.

## Chapter 10: Preparing for Renal Replacement Therapy—Kidney Transplantation, Dialysis, and Dialysis Access

Renal replacement therapy is the term used for the options

of dialysis or kidney transplant.

If you need to choose a form of renal replacement therapy, I strongly encourage you to read the whole chapter.

A preemptive kidney transplant, when available, may be your best option. This means getting a kidney transplant *before* you ever go on dialysis and even before you have an operation on your arm to get a dialysis access.

If you are lucky enough to get a kidney from a related or even an unrelated donor, you are likely to live significantly longer than if you choose dialysis.

Kidney transplants from related and unrelated donors produce the same excellent long-term results.

Your kidney donors can have what is called a minimally invasive surgical procedure to donate their kidney. This surgery is less risky and less invasive than the usual surgical procedure to remove a kidney.

If you do not have a living donor, your next best option is a kidney transplant from someone who dies and donates their kidney, which is a cadaver donor kidney transplant.

The average wait time to get a cadaver kidney is three to five years. Patients with blood type O and B have the longest wait times.

You should start looking for potential kidney donors when your eGFR is around 20 to 30. The workup for you and the donor may take many months to complete.

It is a good idea to get on the cadaver transplant waiting list as early as possible. Most transplant centers will let you get on the list when your eGFR is below 20.

The longer you have been on the waiting list, the higher your priority to get the next available kidney.

You may not benefit by receiving your kidney transplant early, at an eGFR above 10. A delay of the transplant until you have a need for dialysis may be the best approach. This applies to cadaver as well as live donor transplants.

The two choices for dialysis are hemodialysis and peritoneal dialysis. For each modality of dialysis, you can choose to do the treatment at home or in a dialysis unit.

Peritoneal dialysis is the least complicated type of dialysis that you can do at home. It does not require needle sticks. Your kidney team can make a flexible PD schedule that suits you and your lifestyle. You avoid the travel to and from the hemodialysis center. PD can be done every night while you sleep. This daily treatment avoids the "ups and downs" that some patients have with three hemodialysis treatments per week.

Infection is the biggest problem with PD. To avoid infections, you must use good sterile technique.

A disadvantage of PD is the daily treatments versus three times per week for in-center hemodialysis.

Compared with PD, three hemodialysis treatments per week requires stricter limits on your diet and the liquids you take in between treatments.

Low blood pressure during hemodialysis is common. It may decrease blood flow to vital organs, including your heart, as well as your brain and kidneys.

Hemodialysis requires a blood-flow access: a dialysis fistula or a graft. Every time you go on the dialysis machine, at least two large needles are placed in the dialysis access.

Many patients require multiple surgeries to get a working dialysis access. This problem can be decreased if you protect your veins.

One type of access is a fistula, where one of the veins in your arm is connected to an artery. The other type of access is a graft—a tube that goes between the artery and vein in your arm. The fistula is best since it is unlikely to get infected and lasts longer than a graft.

Do not allow needle sticks in the veins of your nondominant arm. For right-handers, this means that you save the veins in the left arm, and for left-handed people, you want to save the veins in your right arm.

After the access surgery, it can take six weeks to three months before the fistula in your arm is ready to use. A graft can provide a usable access in days to weeks.

The last choice for dialysis access is a CVC. The preferable locations for insertion of the CVC are the large veins in your neck. A CVC has the most complications of all access choices. Infections are common and often lead to hospitalizations. In the United States, eight out of ten patients start dialysis with a CVC.

Younger patients who are not in line for a preemptive kidney transplant or home peritoneal dialysis can err on the side of caution and have their dialysis access placed early, around eGFR 15. Hemodialysis is likely in the future, and you are better off getting a working access early to avoid neck catheters (CVC).

Older adults should delay access surgery since death before dialysis is needed is common. If an access is placed too early, some older patients will never use the access. More than half of the new dialysis accesses created in older adults cannot be used. Your kidney team may want to consider a delay in your access until six months before dialysis is expected to start. In some older patients, a CVC may be preferred.

For all patients who face hemodialysis, unless you need emergency dialysis, discuss the option of delaying the dialysis until you have a working dialysis fistula or graft.

# Glossary

**Access**: a device or a construction of blood vessels that allows dialysis to take place, for hemodialysis provides a place to get a patient's blood to flow through the dialysis machine. It can be a fistula, a graft, or a hemodialysis catheter. For peritoneal dialysis, the access point is the abdomen and the access form is a tube-peritoneal catheter.

**Acidosis**: due to buildup of acid or loss of bicarbonate, common with decreased kidney function and called metabolic acidosis; when it is due to accumulation of carbon dioxide in a patient with lung disease, it is called respiratory acidosis.

**Albuminuria**: another name for proteinuria, which refers to the protein albumin in the urine; normally the urine has very small amounts of albumin, and high levels predict a rapid decline in kidney function.

**Alkalosis**: called metabolic alkalosis when too little acid or too much bicarbonate is put in the blood by the kidneys, often occurs with diuretic treatment. If due to rapid breathing, called respiratory alkalosis.

**Acute kidney failure, also called acute kidney injury or AKI**: the worsening of kidney function over a few days or weeks.

**Anemia**: decreased red blood cells or decreased hemoglobin.

**Apnea**: a time interval when you stop breathing, seen with sleep apnea.

**Atherosclerosis**: also called hardening of the arteries, where cholesterol and other substances form a plaque in the arterial wall, blocking the arteries. It is one of the main risks for patients with early-stage CKD.

**Bicarbonate**: an electrolyte that helps keep blood pH from getting too acidic.

**Blood pressure**: the pressure of blood in arteries produced by pumping of the heart. Two numbers of blood pressure are systolic blood pressure—the top number—and diastolic blood pressure—the bottom number.

**Blood sugar**: the level of glucose or sugar in blood together with the A1C level are used to control diabetes.

**Cadaveric kidney donation**: the donation of a kidney by a deceased person to a matched recipient.

**Calcimimetic:** a medication that mimics that action of calcium on the body, which can thereby decrease secretion of PTH.

**Calcitriol:** also called active vitamin D or vitamin D3, produced by normal kidneys.

**Calcium**: a mineral needed for bone health; it may be deposited in the blood vessels in patients with CKD.

**Carbohydrates**: one of the three nutrients. The others are protein and fats.

**Cardiovascular disease**: diseases of the heart and blood vessels common with CKD.

**Cholesterol**: a waxy substance that can be deposited in blood vessels to cause atherosclerosis.

**Chronic kidney disease (CKD)**: decreased kidney function

and/or increased protein in the urine; stages of CKD determined by the level of eGFR and urine protein.

**CKD-MBD**: the abbreviation for the mineral and bone disorder of CKD.

**CHF**: congestive heart failure, a condition where the heart becomes weak and cannot pump enough blood to meet the needs of the body.

**Continuous ambulatory peritoneal dialysis (CAPD)**: a type of peritoneal dialysis (PD) whereby a patient fills their abdomen with peritoneal fluid through the peritoneal catheter. Contrast this to cycler PD, where a machine runs the fluid in and out of the belly, usually while you sleep.

**Contrast-induced kidney failure**: worsening of kidney function after getting intravenous (IV) contrast.

**Coronary heart disease**: hardening of the arteries that supply oxygen to the heart due to plaque buildup from atherosclerosis, one of the risks associated with CKD.

**Creatinine**: a waste product of muscle metabolism that is used to determine estimated kidney function (eGFR), or measured kidney function (twenty-four-hour urine creatinine clearance).

**Creatinine clearance**: a measure of glomerular filtration rate, obtained by dividing the amount of creatinine in a twenty-four-hour urine collection by the serum creatinine.

**Cycler**: a machine that automatically fills the abdomen with new peritoneal dialysis fluid and drains the fluid.

**Diabetic nephropathy**: kidney disease associated with a history of diabetes for more than ten years and elevated urine

187

protein.

**Dialysis**: the process of filtering waste and removing fluid from the blood.

**Diuretic**: medications that get the kidneys to pass more body fluid out in the urine, used to treat blood pressure, CHF, and CKD.

**Edema**: swelling of the feet, ankles, legs. When severe can involve the abdomen and the back.

**Electrolytes**: minerals that can conduct an electrical impulse and help control the body fluids. Major electrolytes are bicarbonate, calcium, chloride, magnesium, phosphate, potassium, and sodium.

**End-stage renal disease**: the term used to describe the point where a patient requires some form of renal replacement therapy—dialysis or kidney transplant; has been used to describe stage 5 CKD.

**Erythropoietin**: a hormone produced by the kidneys that stimulates the production of red blood cells by the bone marrow.

**Fats**: one of the three nutrients. Saturated fats and trans fats can increase atherosclerosis.

**Ferritin level**: a blood test that indicates the amount of iron needed to make red blood cells, is stored in the body.

**Fiber**: a type of carbohydrate that passes through the body undigested. It can help lower glucose levels, decrease colon cancer, helps with constipation.

**Fistula**: a type of dialysis access where a surgeon connects an artery to a vein, usually in the forearm or upper arm. The best type of access for hemodialysis.

**Fluid overload**: the accumulation of body fluids that cause an increase in body weight and edema and can cause shortness of breath. It can be severe in patients who have both kidney and heart disease and can be a reason in some cases to start dialysis.

**Glomerular filtrate**: the filtered liquid that comes out of the glomerular capillaries

**Glomerular filtration rate**: the rate that your kidneys produce the glomerular filtrate every minute.

**Glomerulus**: the tiny blood vessels that are part of the nephron; filters out wastes and toxins.

**Graft**: a type of dialysis access that uses a synthetic tube to connect an artery to a vein.

**Hematuria**: the presence of blood in the urine, usually detected by urinalysis.

**Hematocrit**: the percent of whole blood that is composed of the red blood cells.

**Hemodialysis catheter**: a flexible tube inserted into a vein in your neck or chest that provides access to your bloodstream for dialysis.

**Hemoglobin**: the protein in red blood cells that carries oxygen throughout the body.

**Hemoglobin A1C test**: tells your average level of blood sugar over the past two to three months, also called glycated hemoglobin; nondiabetic people have levels of 6 or less; diabetes can be diagnosed by levels over 6.5.

**HDL**: high-density lipoprotein, a type of cholesterol; was called the good cholesterol, but recent research does not support this idea.

**Home hemodialysis**: dialysis performed at home with the help of a partner, can be three or more times per week.

**Hormone**: a chemical that is produced by the body and released into the bloodstream.

**Hyperglycemia**: abnormally high levels of blood glucose.

**Hyperparathyroidism**: overactivity of parathyroid glands that increase PTH levels in response to CKD, also called secondary hyperparathyroidism.

**Hypertension**: also called high blood pressure; defined by a systolic blood pressure over 140 and/or a diastolic blood pressure over 90.

**Hypoglycemia**: abnormally low level of blood glucose, which may cause clinical symptoms.

**Hypotension**: low levels of blood pressure, usually defined by systolic blood pressure below 90; can cause weakness, dizziness, and decreased blood flow to the heart, brain, and kidneys.

**In-center hemodialysis**: dialysis performed by trained staff in a hospital or freestanding dialysis unit, usually three times per week, three to four hours per treatment.

**Iron saturation**: the amount of iron carried by iron-binding protein. Can indicate a need for more oral or intravenous iron.

**Keto acids**: used as supplements for very-low-protein diets; not proven to benefit most patients with CKD.

**KDIGO**: Kidney Disease Improving Global Outcomes—an international kidney doctor organization dedicated to improving the care and outcomes of patients with kidney disease worldwide through the development and implementation of global clinical practice guidelines.

**Kidney stones**: small mineral deposits in the kidney that can block the ureter.

**Kidney transplant**: a procedure that takes a healthy kidney from a donor who is considered brain dead, or from a relative or friend.

**LDL**: low-density lipoprotein, a type cholesterol, also called bad cholesterol, that carries fat to the walls of blood vessels, which can worsen atherosclerosis.

**Living related donation**: the donation of a kidney by a family member.

**Living unrelated kidney donation**: the donation of a kidney by a friend, or even a stranger.

**Microalbuminuria**: a low level of albumin in the urine.

**Monounsaturated fats**: a type of fat that can improve bad cholesterol levels—found in olive oil, canola oil, peanut oil, sesame oil, and some nuts and seeds.

**Muscle wasting**: a decrease in size of muscles; can lead to lower levels of serum creatinine.

**Nephrologist**: a doctor who specializes in the nonsurgical treatment of kidney disease, as opposed to a urologist, who focuses on surgical interventions for kidney disease.

**Nephron**: the functioning unit of the kidney that removes waste products and excess water and makes urine.

**Nondominant arm**: the arm that a patient uses less frequently; it is usually the arm used for a fistula or a graft.

**Osteoporosis**: a condition where there is decreased calcium in your bones.

**Parathyroidectomy**: the removal of the parathyroid glands.

**Pericarditis**: fluid around the heart, often with chest pain, justifies dialysis if associated with advanced CKD.

**Peritoneal catheter**: a flexible tube inserted into the abdominal wall, then into the abdominal cavity, used to run fluid in and out for peritoneal dialysis.

**Peritoneal dialysis**: a type of dialysis that uses the lining of the abdominal cavity, the peritoneum, to filter waste products out of the blood and remove extra fluid.

**Peritonitis**: an infection of the lining of the peritoneal cavity, called the peritoneum, the major complication of PD.

**Phosphorus binder, or phosphate binder**: a medication that binds dietary phosphorus in the gut.

**Podiatrist**: a health care professional trained in disorders of the feet.

**Polyunsaturated fats**: a type of fat that can improve bad cholesterol levels and decrease atherosclerosis; found in soybean oil, corn oil, sunflower oil, fatty fish, herring, mackerel, and salmon.

**Potassium**: a mineral needed for healthy heart, muscle, and nerve function; levels are controlled by the kidneys; high hyperkalemia and low hypokalemia levels can cause weakness, numbness, tingling, and dangerous heart rhythms.

**Proteinuria**: the presence of protein in the urine, usually detected by urinalysis.

**PTH**: parathyroid hormone, a hormone secreted by the parathyroid glands that regulates calcium and phosphorus levels in the body, acts on bones and kidneys.

**Red blood cells**: the part of the blood that contains hemoglobin, which carries oxygen to all the organs of the body.

**Renal replacement therapy**: another name for dialysis and transplant.

**Residual kidney function**: a patient's own kidney function that is present at the time they are considered for dialysis; even small amounts have survival and quality-of-life benefits.

**Sleep apnea**: an abnormal sleep pattern; patients intermittently stop breathing for several seconds or longer; may contribute to elevated blood pressure.

**Sodium**: a mineral that determines the volume of body fluids; retention by the kidneys can cause edema.

**Spot urine for protein**: a tiny sample of your urine that estimates your twenty-four-hour urine protein.

**Transplant list**: a list of patients who have completed the transplant workup and are waiting for a cadaver kidney transplant.

**Ureters**: two thin tubes that connect the kidneys to the bladder.

**Urethra**: the tube that allows urine to pass out of the body.

**Urinalysis**: a range of tests done on a urine sample to detect glucose, protein, blood, and blood cells.

**Urologist**: a surgeon who specializes in diseases of the kidney's ureters and bladder.

**Vegan diet**: a diet that excludes all meat and dairy products.

**Vegetarian diet**: a diet that focuses on plant foods, fruits, vegetables, beans, grains, seeds, nuts, and does not include meat or seafood; some vegetarians eat dairy products and fish.

**Vein mapping**: a noninvasive ultrasound technique that helps to determine which veins are suitable for an AV access.

# References

## Introduction

Debelle, Frédéric D., Jean-Louis Vanherweghem, and Joëlle L. Nortier. "Aristolochic Acid Nephropathy: A Worldwide Problem." *Kidney International* 74, no. 2 (July 2008): 158–69. https://doi.org/10.1038/ki.2008.129.

Klahr, Saulo, Andrew S. Levey, Gerald J. Beck, Arlene W. Caggiula, Lawrence Hunsicker, John W. Kusek, and Gary Striker. "The Effects of Dietary Protein Restriction and Blood-Pressure Control on the Progression of Chronic Renal Disease." Modification of Diet in Renal Disease Study Group. *New England Journal of Medicine* 330, no. 13 (March 31, 1994): 877–84. https://doi.org/10.1056/nejm199403313301301.

Li, Xiao-Feng, Jing Xu, Ling-Jiao Liu, Fang Wang, Sheng-Lin He, Ya Su, and Chun-Ping Dong. "Efficacy of Low-Protein Diet in Diabetic Nephropathy: a Meta-Analysis of Randomized Controlled Trials." *Lipids in Health and Disease* 18, no. 1 (January 2019). https://doi.org/10.1186/s12944-019-1007-6.

Massy, Ziad A., Jean Ferrières, Eric Bruckert, Céline Lange,

Sophie Liabeuf, Maja Velkovski-Rouyer, Bénédicte Stengel, et al. "Achievement of Low-Density Lipoprotein Cholesterol Targets in CKD." *Kidney International Reports* 4, no. 11 (2019): 1546–54. https://doi.org/10.1016/j.ekir.2019.07.014.

Menon, Vandana, Joel D. Kopple, Xuelei Wang, Gerald J. Beck, Allan J. Collins, John W. Kusek, Tom Greene, Andrew S. Levey, and Mark J. Sarnak. "Effect of a Very Low-Protein Diet on Outcomes: Long-Term Follow-up of the Modification of Diet in Renal Disease (MDRD) Study." *American Journal of Kidney Diseases* 53, no. 2 (February 2009): 208–17. https://doi.org/10.1053/j.ajkd.2008.08.009.

Tummalapalli, Sri Lekha, Neil R. Powe, and Salomeh Keyhani. "Trends in Quality of Care for Patients with CKD in the United States." Clinical Journal of the American Society of Nephrology 14, no. 8 (August 7, 2019): 1142–50. https://doi.org/10.2215/cjn.00060119.

## Chapter 1

Bauer, Carolyn, Michal L. Melamed, and Thomas H. Hostetter. "Staging of Chronic Kidney Disease: Time for a Course Correction." *Journal of the American Society of Nephrology* 19, no. 5 (May 2, 2008): 844–46. https://doi.org/10.1681/asn.2008010110.

Beddhu, S., M. H. Samore , M. S. Roberts, G. J. Stoddard, L. M. Pappas, and A. K. Cheung. "Creatinine Production, Nutrition, and

Glomerular Filtration Rate Estimation." *Journal of the American Society of Nephrology* 14, no. 4 (January 2003): 1000–1005. https://doi.org/10.1097/01.asn.0000057856.88335.dd.

"Summary of Recommendation Statements." *Kidney International Supplements* 3, no. 1 (2013): 5–14. https://doi.org/10.1038/kisup.2012.77.

Eckardt, K. U., N. Bansal, J. Coresh, and M. Evans. "Improving the Prognosis of Patients with Severely Decreased Glomerular Filtration Rate (CKD G4D): Conclusions from a Kidney Disease: Improving Global Outcomes (KDIGO) Controversies Conference." *Kidney International* 93, no. 6 (June 2018): 1281–92.

Qaseem, Amir, Robert H. Hopkins, Donna E. Sweet, Melissa Starkey, and Paul Shekelle. "Screening, Monitoring, and Treatment of Stage 1 to 3 Chronic Kidney Disease: A Clinical Practice Guideline From the Clinical Guidelines Committee of the American College of Physicians." Annals of Internal Medicine 159, no. 12 (December 17, 2013): 835–47. https://doi.org/10.7326/0003-4819-159-12-201312170-00726.

Rayner, Hugh C., and Steven J. Rosansky. "The Estimated Glomerular Filtration Rate Graph: Another Tool in the Management of Patients with Advanced Chronic Kidney Disease." *Kidney International* 94, no. 1 (July 2018): 222. https://doi.org/10.1016/j.kint.2018.04.016.

Rosansky, Steven J. "Renal Function Trajectory Is More Important than Chronic Kidney Disease Stage for Managing Patients with Chronic Kidney Disease." American Journal of Nephrology 36, no. 1 (June 13, 2012): 1–10. https://doi.org/10.1159/000339327.

Chapter 2

Ahmad, Iram, Leila R. Zelnick, Zona Batacchi, Nicole Robinson, Ashveena Dighe, Jo-Anne E. Manski-Nankervis, John Furler, et al. "Hypoglycemia in People with Type 2 Diabetes and CKD." Clinical Journal of the American Society of Nephrology 14, no. 6 (June 7, 2019): 844–53. https://doi.org/10.2215/cjn.11650918.

Banerjee, Tanushree, Deidra C. Crews, Delphine S. Tuot, Meda E. Pavkov, Nilka Rios Burrows, Austin G. Stack, Rajiv Saran, et al. "Poor Accordance to a DASH Dietary Pattern Is Associated with Higher Risk of ESRD among Adults with Moderate Chronic Kidney Disease and Hypertension." Kidney International 95, no. 6 (June 2019): 1433–42. https://doi.org/10.1016/j.kint.2018.12.027.

Coresh, J., T. C. Turin, K. Matsushita, Y. Sang, S. H. Ballew, and L. J. Appel. "Decline in Estimated Glomerular Filtration Rate and Subsequent Risk of End-Stage Renal Disease and Mortality." JAMA 311, no. 24 (June 25, 2014): 2518–31.

Delles, Christian, and Gemma Currie. "Proteinuria and Its Relation to Cardiovascular Disease." International Journal of

*Nephrology and Renovascular Disease* 7 (December 21, 2013): 13–24. https://doi.org/10.2147/ijnrd.s40522.

Hemmelgarn, Brenda R., Braden J. Manns, Anita Lloyd, Matthew T. James, Scott Klarenbach, Robert R. Quinn, Natasha Wiebe, et al. "Relation Between Kidney Function, Proteinuria, and Adverse Outcomes." *JAMA* 303, no. 5 (March 2010): 423–429. https://doi.org/10.1001/jama.2010.39.

"KDIGO Clinical Practice Guideline for Lipid Management in Chronic Kidney Disease." *Kidney International Supplements* 3, no. 3 (November 2013): .

Kwon, Yeongkeun, Kyungdo Han, Yang Hyun Kim, Sungsoo Park, Do Hoon Kim, Yong Kyun Roh, Yong-Gyu Park, and Kyung-Hwan Cho. "Dipstick Proteinuria Predicts All-Cause Mortality in General Population: A Study of 17 Million Korean Adults." *Plos One* 13, no. 6 (June 28, 2018). https://doi.org/10.1371/journal.pone.0199913.

Levy, Jeremy. "Proteinuria, Renal Impairment, and Death: If reducing proteinuria improves cardiovascular outcomes, urine dipstick testing will become crucial in hypertension." *BMJ* 332, no. 7555 (June 17, 2006): 1402–3. https://doi.org/10.1136/bmj.332.7555.1402.

Li, Yanping, An Pan, Dong D. Wang, Xiaoran Liu, Klodian Dhana, Oscar H. Franco, Stephen Kaptoge, et al. "Impact of Healthy Lifestyle Factors on Life Expectancies in the US Population." *Circulation* 138, no. 4 (July 24, 2018): 345–55. https://doi.org/10.1161/circulationaha.117.032047.

Nagata, M., T. Ninomiya, Y. Kiyohara, Y. Murakami, F. Irie, T. Sairenchi, K. Miura, T. Okamura, and H. Ueshima. "Prediction of Cardiovascular Disease Mortality by Proteinuria and Reduced Kidney Function: Pooled Analysis of 39,000 Individuals From 7 Cohort Studies in Japan." *American Journal of Epidemiology* 178, no. 1 (July 1, 2013): 1–11. https://doi.org/10.1093/aje/kws447.

Olechnowicz-Tietz, Sylwia, Anna Gluba, Anna Paradowska, Maciej Banach, and Jacek Rysz. "The Risk of Atherosclerosis in Patients with Chronic Kidney Disease." *International Urology and Nephrology* 45, no. 6 (March 13, 2013): 1605–12. https://doi.org/10.1007/s11255-013-0407-1.

Sun, Yang, Anxin Wang, Xiaoxue Liu, Zhaoping Su, Junjuan Li, Yanxia Luo, Shuohua Chen, et al. "Changes in Proteinuria on the Risk of All-Cause Mortality in People with Diabetes or Prediabetes: A Prospective Cohort Study." *Journal of Diabetes Research* 2017 (September 27, 2017): 1–7. https://doi.org/10.1155/2017/8368513.

## Chapter 3

Bach, Katrina E., Jaimon T. Kelly, Suetonia C. Palmer, Saman Khalesi, Giovanni F. M. Strippoli, and Katrina L.

Campbell. "Healthy Dietary Patterns and Incidence of CKD: A Meta-Analysis of Cohort Studies." *Clinical Journal of the American Society of Nephrology* 14, no. 10 (October 7, 2019): 1441–49. https://doi.org/10.2215/cjn.00530119.

Gabardi, Steven, Kristin Munz, and Catherine Ulbricht. "A Review of Dietary Supplement–Induced Renal Dysfunction." *Clinical Journal of the American Society of Nephrology* 2, no. 4 (July 2007): 757–65. https://doi.org/10.2215/cjn.00500107.

Hruby, Adela, Shivani Sahni, Douglas Bolster, and Paul F. Jacques. "Protein Intake and Functional Integrity in Aging: The Framingham Heart Study Offspring." *The Journals of Gerontology: Series A* 75, no. 1 (September 24, 2018): 123–30. https://doi.org/10.1093/gerona/gly201.

Hu, Emily A., and Casey M. Rebholz. "Can Dietary Patterns Modify Risk for CKD?" *Clinical Journal of the American Society of Nephrology* 14, no. 10 (October 7, 2019): 1419–20. https://doi.org/10.2215/cjn.09440819.

Lennon, Michael J. "Diet Patterns and Kidney Disease." *Clinical Journal of the American Society of Nephrology* 14, no. 10 (September, 24, 2019): 1417–18. https://doi.org/10.2215/cjn.09660819.

Steven Rosansky

## Chapter 4

Clark, Edward G., and Swapnil Hiremath. "Progressively Earlier Initiation of Renal Replacement Therapy for Acute Kidney Injury Is Unwarranted and Potentially Harmful." *Blood Purification* 41, no. 1–3 (March 2016): 159–65. https://doi.org/10.1159/000441263.

"KDIGO Clinical Practice Guideline for Acute Kidney Injury Prevention and Treatment of AKI." *Kidney International Supplements 2*, no. 7 (March 2012): .

Ku, Elaine, Joachim H. Ix, Kenneth Jamerson, Navdeep Tangri, Feng Lin, Jennifer Gassman, Miroslaw Smogorzewski, and Mark J. Sarnak. "Acute Declines in Renal Function during Intensive BP Lowering and Long-Term Risk of Death." *Journal of the American Society of Nephrology* 29, no. 9 (September 2018): 2401–8. https://doi.org/10.1681/asn.2018040365.

Lee, Benjamin J., Chi-Yuan Hsu, Rishi Parikh, Charles E. Mcculloch, Thida C. Tan, Kathleen D. Liu, Raymond K. Hsu, Leonid Pravoverov, Sijie Zheng, and Alan S. Go. "Predicting Renal Recovery After Dialysis-Requiring Acute Kidney Injury." *Kidney International Reports* 4, no. 4 (January 28, 2019): 571–81. https://doi.org/10.1016/j.ekir.2019.01.015.

McCallum, Wendy, Hocine Tighiouart, Elaine Ku, Deeb Salem, and Mark J. Sarnak. "Acute Declines in Estimated Glomerular

Filtration Rate on Enalapril and Mortality and Cardiovascular Outcomes in Patients with Heart Failure with Reduced Ejection Fraction." *Kidney International* 96, no. 5 (June 11, 2019): 1185–94. https://doi.org/10.1016/j.kint.2019.05.019.

Prowle, John R., and Andrew Davenport. "Does Early-Start Renal Replacement Therapy Improve Outcomes for Patients with Acute Kidney Injury?" *Kidney International* 88, no. 4 (October 2015): 670–73. https://doi.org/10.1038/ki.2015.225.

Rosansky, Steven. "Is Hypertension Overtreatment a Silent Epidemic?" *Archives of Internal Medicine* 172, no. 22 (December 10, 2012): 1769. https://doi.org/10.1001/2013.jamainternmed.96.

Seabra, Victor F., Ethan M. Balk, Orfeas Liangos, Marie Anne Sosa, Miguel Cendoroglo, and Bertrand L. Jaber. "Timing of Renal Replacement Therapy Initiation in Acute Renal Failure: A Meta-Analysis." *American Journal of Kidney Diseases* 52, no. 2 (August 2008): 272–84. https://doi.org/10.1053/j.ajkd.2008.02.371.

## Chapter 5

Al-Aly, Ziyad, Angelique Zeringue, John Fu, Michael I. Rauchman, Jay R. McDonald, Tarek M. El-Achkar, Sumitra Balasubramanian, et al. "Rate of Kidney Function Decline Associates with Mortality." *Journal of the American Society of Nephrology* 21, no. 10 (October 2010): 1961–69. https://doi.

Steven Rosansky

org/10.1681/asn.2009121210.

American Diabetes Association. "Glycemic Targets: Standards of Medical Care in Diabetes—2019." *Diabetes Care* 42, Supplement 1 (January 2019): S61–S70. https://doi.org/10.2337/dc19-s006.

Bakris, George. "Chronic Kidney Disease: Optimal Blood Pressure for Kidney Disease—Lower Is Not Better." *Nature Reviews Nephrology* 9, no. 11 (November 2013): 634–5. doi:10.1038/nrneph.2013.206.

Chang, Alex R., Meghan Lóser, Rakesh Malhotra, and Lawrence J. Appel. "Blood Pressure Goals in Patients with CKD: A Review of Evidence and Guidelines." *Clinical Journal of the American Society of Nephrology* 14, no. 5 (January 7, 2019): 161-169. https://doi.org/10.2215/cjn.07440618.

Chang, Tara I., and Mark J. Sarnak. "Intensive Blood Pressure Targets and Kidney Disease." *Clinical Journal of the American Society of Nephrology* 13, no. 10 (October 8, 2018): 1575–77.

Cheung, Alfred K., Tara I. Chang, William C. Cushman, Susan L. Furth, Joachim H. Ix, Roberto Pecoits-Filho, Vlado Perkovic, et al. "Blood Pressure in Chronic Kidney Disease: Conclusions from a Kidney Disease: Improving Global Outcomes (KDIGO) Controversies Conference." *Kidney International* 95, no. 5 (May 2019): 1027–36.

Clark, William F., Jessica M. Sontrop, Shih-Han Huang, Kerri Gallo, Louise Moist, Andrew A. House, Meaghan S. Cuerden, et al. "Effect of Coaching to Increase Water Intake on Kidney Function Decline in Adults With Chronic Kidney Disease: The CKD WIT Randomized Clinical Trial." *Journal of the American Medical Association* 319, no. 18 (May 8, 2018): 1870–9. doi:10.1001/jama.2018.4930.

Coresh, Josef, Andrew S. Levey. "A Combination of Change in Albuminuria and GFR as a Surrogate End Point for Progression of CKD." *Clinical Journal of the American Society of Nephrology* 14, no. 6 (Jun 7, 2019): 792–4. doi:10.2215/CJN.04160419.

Garneata, Liliana, Alexandra Stancu, Diana Dragomir, Gabriel Stefan, and Gabriel Mircescu. "Ketoanalogue-Supplemented Vegetarian Very Low–Protein Diet and CKD Progression." *Journal of the American Society of Nephrology* 27, no. 7 (July 2016): 2164–76. https://doi.org/10.1681/asn.2015040369.

Hruby, Adela, Shivani Sahni, Douglas Bolster, and Paul F. Jacques. "Protein Intake and Functional Integrity in Aging: The Framingham Heart Study Offspring." *The Journals of Gerontology: Series A* 75, no. 1 (September 24, 2018): 123–30. https://doi.org/10.1093/gerona/gly201.

Kim, Hyunju, Laura E. Caulfield, Vanessa Garcia-Larsen, Lyn M. Steffen, Morgan E. Grams, Josef Coresh, and Casey M. Rebholz. "Plant-Based Diets and Incident CKD and Kidney

Function." *Clinical Journal of the American Society of Nephrology* 14, no. 5 (May 2019): 682–91. https://doi.org/10.2215/cjn.12391018

Ko, Gang Jee, Yoshitsugu Obi, Amanda R. Tortorici, and Kamyar Kalantar-Zadeh. "Dietary Protein Intake and Chronic Kidney Disease." *Current Opinion in Clinical Nutrition and Metabolic Care* 20, no. 1 (January 2017): 77–85. https://doi.org/10.1097/MCO.0000000000000342.

Marcum Zachary A., Emily P. Peron, and Joseph T. Hanlon. "Recognizing the Risks of Chronic Nonsteroidal Anti-Inflammatory Drug Use in Older Adults." *Annals of Long-term Care* 18, no. 9 (September 2012): 24–27. https://doi.org/10.1007/978-94-007-5061-6_18.

Metzger, Marie, Wen Lun Yuan, Jean-Philippe Haymann, Martin Flamant, Pascal Houillier, Eric Thervet, Jean-Jacques Boffa, et al. "Association of a Low-Protein Diet With Slower Progression of CKD." Kidney Int Rep (2018) 3, 105–114; http://dx.doi.org/10.1016/j.ekir.2017.08.010

Murphy, Daniel P., Paul E. Drawz, and Robert N. Foley. "Trends in Angiotensin-Converting Enzyme Inhibitor and Angiotensin II Receptor Blocker Use among Those with Impaired Kidney Function in the United States." *Journal of the American Society of Nephrology* 30, no. 7 (June 2019): 1314–21. https://doi:10.1681/ASN.2018100971

Navaneethan, Sankar D., Jun Shao, Jerry Buysse, and David A. Bushinsky. "Effects of Treatment of Metabolic Acidosis in CKD: A Systematic Review and Meta-Analysis." *Clinical Journal of the American Society of Nephrology* 14, no. 7 (2019): 1011–20. https://doi.org/10.2215/cjn.13091118.

Ohkuma, Toshiaki, Min Jun, John Chalmers, Mark E. Cooper, Pavel Hamet, Stephen Harrap, Sophia Zoungas, Vlado Perkovic, Mark Woodward, et al. "Combination of Changes in Estimated GFR and Albuminuria and the Risk of Major Clinical Outcomes." *Clinical Journal of the American Society of Nephrology* 14, no. 6 (Jun 7, 2019): 862–72. https://doi:10.2215/CJN.13391118.

Satirapoj, Bancha, Peerapong Vongwattana, and Ouppatham Supasyndh. "Very Low Protein Diet plus Ketoacid Analogs of Essential Amino Acids Supplement to Retard Chronic Kidney Disease Progression." Kidney Research and Clinical Practice 37, no. 4 (December 31, 2018): 384–92. https://doi.org/10.23876/j.krcp.18.0055.

Sinha, Arjun D., and Rajiv Agarwal. "Clinical Pharmacology of Antihypertensive Therapy for the Treatment of Hypertension in CKD." *Clinical Journal of the American Society of Nephrology* 14, no. 5 (May 7, 2019): 757–64. https://doi.org/10.2215/cjn.04330418.

Smith, Margaret, William G. Herrington, Misghina

Weldegiorgis, F. D. Richard Hobbs, Clare Bankhead, and Mark Woodward. "Change in Albuminuria and Risk of Renal and Cardiovascular Outcomes: Natural Variation Should Be Taken into Account." *Kidney International Reports* 3, no. 4 (July 2018): 939–49. https://doi.org/10.1016/j.ekir.2018.04.004.

Sun, Jing, Hongjun Sun, Meiyu Cui, Zhijian Sun, Wenyue Li, Jianxin Wei, and Shuhua Zhou. "The Use of Anti-Ulcer Agents and the Risk of Chronic Kidney Disease: A Meta-Analysis." *International Urology and Nephrology* 50, no. 10 (June 13, 2018): 1835–43. https://doi.org/10.1007/s11255-018-1908-8.

Yan, Bingjuan, Xiaole Su, Boyang Xu, Xi Qiao, and Lihua Wang. "Effect of Diet Protein Restriction on Progression of Chronic Kidney Disease: A Systematic Review and Meta-Analysis." *Plos One* 13, no. 11 (November 7, 2018): . https://doi.org/10.1371/journal.pone.0206134.

**Chapter 6**

Grams, Morgan E., Yingying Sang, Shoshana H. Ballew, Juan Jesus Carrero, Ognjenka Djurdjev, et al. "Predicting Timing of Clinical Outcomes in Patients with Chronic Kidney Disease and Severely Decreased Glomerular Filtration Rate." *Kidney International* 93, no. 6 (June 2018): 1442–51. https://doi.org/10.1016/j.kint.2018.01.009.

O'Hare, Ann. M., A. I. Choi, D. Bertenthal, P. Bacchetti, A. X.

Garg, J. S. Kaufman, et al. "Age Affects Outcomes in Chronic Kidney Disease. *Journal of the American Society of Nephrology* 18, no. 10 (October 2007): 2758–2765. https://doi.org/10.1681/ASN.2007040422

O'Hare, Ann M., Adam Batten, Nilka Ríos Burrows, Meda E. Pavkov, Leslie Taylor, Indra Gupta, Jeff Todd-Stenberg, et al. "Trajectories of Kidney Function Decline in the 2 Years Before Initiation of Long-Term Dialysis." *American Journal of Kidney Diseases* 59, no. 4 (April 2012): 513–22. https://doi.org/10.1053/j.ajkd.2011.11.044.

Potok, O. Alison, Hoang Anh Nguyen, Joseph A. Abdelmalek, Tomasz Beben, Tyler B. Woodell, and Dena E. Rifkin. "Patients,' Nephrologists,' and Predicted Estimations of ESKD Risk Compared with 2-Year Incidence of ESKD." *Clinical Journal of the American Society of Nephrology* 14, no. 2 (February 2019): 206–12. https://doi.org/10.2215/cjn.07970718.

Ravani, Pietro, Marta Fiocco, Ping Liu, Robert R. Quinn, Brenda Hemmelgarn, Matthew James, Ngan Lam, Braden Manns, Matthew J. Oliver, et al. "Influence of Mortality on Estimating t he Risk of Kidney Failure in People with Stage 4 Chronic Kidney Disease." *Journal of the American Society of Nephrology* 30, no. 11 (September 20, 2019): 2219–2227. https://doi.org/10.1681/ASN.2019060640

Stevens, Paul. E., and Christopher. K. T. Farmer. "Chronic

Kidney Disease and Life Expectancy." *Nephrology Dialysis Transplantation* 27, no. 8 (August 2012): 3014–15. https://doi.org/10.1093/ndt/gfs309.

Tangri, Navdeep, Morgan E. Grams, Andrew S. Levey, Josef Coresh, Lawrence J. Appel, Brad C. Astor, Gabriel Chodick, et al. "Multinational Assessment of Accuracy of Equations for Predicting Risk of Kidney Failure: A Meta-analysis." *JAMA* 315, no. 2 (2016): 164–174. https://doi.org/10.1001/jama.2015.18202.

Turin, Tanvir Chowdhury, Marcello Tonelli, Braden J. Manns, Pietro Ravani, Sofia B. Ahmed, and Brenda R. Hemmelgarn. "Chronic Kidney Disease and Life Expectancy." *Nephrology Dialysis Transplantation* 27, no. 8 (August 2012): 3182–86. https://doi.org/10.1093/ndt/gfs052.

**Chapter 7**

Chen, Wei, and Matthew K. Abramowitz. "Treatment of Metabolic Acidosis in Patients With CKD." *American Journal of Kidney Diseases* 63, no. 2 (February 2014): 311–17. https://doi.org/10.1053/j.ajkd.2013.06.017.

Pitt, Bertram, and George L. Bakris. "New Potassium Binders for the Treatment of Hyperkalemia." *Hypertension* 66, no. 4 (August 24, 2015): 731–38. https://doi.org/10.1161/hypertensionaha.115.04889.

Souto, Gema, Cristóbal Donapetry, Jesús Calviño, and Maria M. Adeva. "Metabolic Acidosis-Induced Insulin Resistance and Cardiovascular Risk." *Metabolic Syndrome and Related Disorders* 9, no. 4 (July 25, 2011): 247–53. https://doi.org/10.1089/met.2010.0108.

Spinowitz, Bruce S., Steven Fishbane, Pablo E. Pergola, Simon D. Roger, Edgar V. Lerma, Javed Butler, Stephan Von Haehling, et al. "Sodium Zirconium Cyclosilicate among Individuals with Hyperkalemia." *Clinical Journal of the American Society of Nephrology* 14, no. 6 (June 7, 2019): 798–809. https://doi.org/10.2215/cjn.12651018.

**Chapter 8**

Barreto, Fellype Carvalho, Daniela Veit Barreto, Ziad A. Massy, and Tilman B. Drüeke. "Strategies for Phosphate Control in Patients With CKD." *Kidney International Reports* 4, no. 8 (June 20, 2019): 1043–56. https://doi.org/10.1016/j.ekir.2019.06.002.

"KDIGO Clinical Practice Guideline for Anemia in Chronic Kidney Disease." *Kidney International Supplements* 2, no. 4 (August 2012): .

Ketteler, Markus, Geoffrey A. Block, Pieter Evenepoel, Masafumi Fukagawa, Charles A. Herzog, Linda McCann, Sharon M. Moe, et al. "Diagnosis, Evaluation, Prevention, and Treatment of Chronic Kidney Disease—Mineral and Bone Disorder: Synopsis of the Kidney Disease: Improving Global Outcomes 2017 Clinical Practice Guideline Update." *Annals of Internal Medicine* 168, no. 6 (March 20, 2018): 422–30. https://doi.org/10.7326/m17-2640.

Melamed, Michal L., Rupinder Singh Buttar, and Maria Coco. "CKD-Mineral Bone Disorder in Stage 4 and 5 CKD: What We Know Today?" *Advances in Chronic Kidney Disease* 23, no. 4 (July 2016): 262–69. https://doi.org/10.1053/j.ackd.2016.03.008.

Negrea, Lavinia. "Active Vitamin D in Chronic Kidney Disease: Getting Right Back Where We Started from?" *Kidney Diseases* 5, no. 2 (March 2019): 59–68. https://doi.org/10.1159/000495138.

Tonelli, Marcello. "Serum Phosphorus in People with Chronic Kidney Disease: You Are What You Eat." *Kidney International* 84, no. 5 (November 2013): 871–73. https://doi.org/10.1038/ki.2013.258.

Whittaker, Chanel F., Margaret A. Miklich, Roshni S. Patel, and Jeffrey C. Fink. "Medication Safety Principles and Practice in CKD." *Clinical Journal of the American Society of Nephrology* 13, no. 11 (November 7, 2018): 1738–46. https://doi.org/10.2215/cjn.00580118.

**Chapter 9**

Assa, Solmaz, Yoran M. Hummel, Adriaan A. Voors, Johanna Kuipers, Ralf Westerhuis, Paul E. De Jong, and Casper F. M.

Franssen. "Hemodialysis-Induced Regional Left Ventricular Systolic Dysfunction: Prevalence, Patient and Dialysis Treatment-Related Factors, and Prognostic Significance." *Clinical Journal of the American Society of Nephrology* 7, no. 10 (July 19, 2012): 1615–23. https://doi.org/10.2215/cjn.00850112.

Berns, Jeffrey S., Tonya L. Saffer, and Eugene Lin. "Addressing Financial Disincentives to Improve CKD Care." *Journal of the American Society of Nephrology* 29, no. 11 (October 2018): 2610–12. https://doi.org/10.1681/asn.2018040438.

Bleyer, Anthony J., and Amret Hawfield. "Modifiable Risk Factors for Sudden Death in Dialysis Patients." *Nature Reviews Nephrology* 8, no. 6 (May 1, 2012): 323–24. https://doi.org/10.1038/nrneph.2012.84.

Brimble, K. Scott, Rajnish Mehrotra, Marcello Tonelli, Carmel M. Hawley, Clare Castledine, Stephen P. McDonald, Vicki Levidiotis, et al. "Estimated GFR Reporting Influences Recommendations for Dialysis Initiation." *Journal of the American Society of Nephrology* 24, no. 11 (August 2013): 1737–42. https://doi.org/10.1681/asn.2013010035.

Burton, J. O., H. J. Jefferies, N. M. Selby, C. W. McIntyre. "Hemodialysis-Induced Cardiac Injury: Determinants and Associated Outcomes." *Clinical Journal of the American Society of Nephrology* 4, no. 5 (May 2009): 914–920. https://doi.org/10.2215/CJN.03900808.

Steven Rosansky

Cooper, Bruce A., Pauline Branley, Liliana Bulfone, John F. Collins, Jonathan C. Craig, Margaret B. Fraenkel, Anthony Harris, et al. "A Randomized, Controlled Trial of Early versus Late Initiation of Dialysis." *New England Journal of Medicine* 363, no. 7 (August 12, 2010): 609–19. https://doi.org/10.1056/nejmoa1000552.

Crews, Deidra C., Bernard G. Jaar, Laura C. Plantinga, Hania S. Kassem, Nancy E. Fink, and Neil R. Powe. "Inpatient Hemodialysis Initiation: Reasons, Risk Factors and Outcomes." *Nephron Clinical Practice* 114, no. 1 (February 2010): c19–c28. https://doi.org/10.1159/000245066.

Di Micco, Lucia, Serena Torraca, Andrea Pota, Daniela Di Giuseppe, Antonio Pisani, Letizia Spinelli, Simona De Portu, Massimo Sabbatini, Lorenzo Mantovani, and Bruno Cianciaruso. "Setting Dialysis Start at 6.0 Ml/Min/1.73 m2 EGFR—a Study on Safety, Quality of Life, and Economic Impact." *Nephrology Dialysis Transplantation* 24, no. 11 (November 2009): 3434–40. https://doi.org/10.1093/ndt/gfp281.

Ellwood, Amanda D., S. Vanita Jassal, Rita S. Suri, William F. Clark, Yingo Na, and Louise M. Moist. "Early Dialysis Initiation and Rates and Timing of Withdrawal From Dialysis in Canada." *Clinical Journal of the American Society of Nephrology* 8, no. 2 (February 7, 2013): 265–70. https://doi.org/10.2215/cjn.01000112.

House, A., C. Wanner, M. J. Sarnak. "Heart Failure in Chronic Kidney Disease: Conclusions from a Kidney Disease: Improving Global Outcomes (KDIGO) Controversies Conference." *Kidney International* 95, no. 6 (June 2019): 1304–1317.

Khan, Yusra Habib, Azmi Sarriff, Azreen Syazril Adnan, Amer Hayat Khan, and Tauqeer Hussain Mallhi. "Chronic Kidney Disease, Fluid Overload and Diuretics: A Complicated Triangle." *Plos One* 11, no.7 (July 21, 2016): . https://doi. org/10.1371/journal.pone.0159335.

McIntyre, Christopher W., and Steven J. Rosansky. "Starting Dialysis Is Dangerous: How Do We Balance the Risk?" *Kidney International* 82, no. 4 (August 2012): 382–87. https://doi. org/10.1038/ki.2012.133.

National Kidney Foundation, Transl. Dmytro D. Ivanov. "KDOQI Clinical Practice Guideline for Hemodialysis Adequacy: 2015 Update." *American Journal of Kidney Diseases* 66, no. 5 (November 2015): 884–930.

Okuda, Yusuke, Melissa Soohoo, Ying Tang, Yoshitsugu Obi, Marciana Laster, Connie M. Rhee, Elani Streja, and Kamyar Kalantar-Zadeh. "Estimated GFR at Dialysis Initiation and Mortality in Children and Adolescents." *American Journal of Kidney Diseases* 73, no. 6: 797–805. https://doi.org/10.1053/j. ajkd.2018.12.038.

Steven Rosansky

Perl, Jeffrey, and Joanne M. Bargman. "The Importance of Residual Kidney Function for Patients on Dialysis: A Critical Review." *American Journal of Kidney Diseases* 53, no. 6 (June 2009): 1068–81. https://doi.org/10.1053/j.ajkd.2009.02.012.

Rosansky, Steven J., G. Cancarini, William F. Clark, Paul Eggers, M. Germaine, Richard Glassock, et al. "Dialysis Initiation: What's the Rush?" *Seminars in Dialysis* 26, no. 6 (Nov-Dec 2013): 650–57.

Rosansky, Steven J., Mae Thamer, Fergus Caskey, Cécile Couchoud, Stephen P. McDonald, and Louise Moist. "A Comparison of Predialysis Estimated Glomerular Filtration Rate in the US, Canada, France, Australia, and the UK between 2005 and 2015." *Kidney International* 95, no. 5 (May 2019): 1273. https://doi.org/10.1016/j.kint.2019.02.008.

Rosansky, Steven J., Paul Eggers, Kirby Jackson, Richard J. Glassock, and William F. Clark. "Early Start of Hemodialysis May Be Harmful." *Archives of Internal Medicine* 171, no. 5 (March 14, 2011). https://doi.org/10.1001/archinternmed.2010.415.

Rosansky, Steven J., Richard J. Glassock, and William F. Clark. "Early Start of Dialysis: A Critical Review." *Clinical Journal of the American Society of Nephrology* 6, no. 5 (May 2011): 1222–28. https://doi.org/10.2215/cjn.09301010.

Rosansky, Steven J., William F. Clark, Paul Eggers, and Richard J. Glassock. "Initiation of Dialysis at Higher GFRs: Is the Apparent

Rising Tide of Early Dialysis Harmful or Helpful?" *Kidney International* 76, no. 3 (August 2009): 257–61. https://doi.org/10.1038/ki.2009.161.

Susantitaphong, Paweena, Sarah Altamimi, Motaz Ashkar, Ethan M. Balk, Vianda S. Stel, Seth Wright, and Bertrand L. Jaber. "GFR at Initiation of Dialysis and Mortality in CKD: A Meta-Analysis." *American Journal of Kidney Diseases* 59, no. 6 (June 2012): 829–40. https://doi.org/10.1053/j.ajkd.2012.01.015.

Vanholder, Raymond, Nic Veys, and Wim Van Biesen. "Long Weekend Hemodialysis Intervals—Killing Fields?" *Nature Reviews Nephrology* 8, no. 1 (November 22, 2011): 5–6. https://doi.org/10.1038/nrneph.2011.192.

Wright, Seth, Dalia Klausner, Bradley Baird, Mark E. Williams, Theodore Steinman, Hongying Tang, Regina Ragasa, Alexander S. Goldfard-Rumyantzev: "Timing of Dialysis Initiation and Survival in ESRD." *Clinical Journal of the American Society of Nephrology* 5, no. 10 (October 2010): 1828–1835.

**Chapter 10**

Abel, Daniel L. "Functioning on Dialysis: An Oxymoron?" *Clinical Journal of the American Society of Nephrology* 14, no. 7 (July 5, 2019): 963–64. https://doi.org/10.2215/cjn.05870519.

Agarwal, Anil K., Nabil J. Haddad, Tushar J. Vachharajani, and

Arif Asif. "Innovations in Vascular Access for Hemodialysis." *Kidney International* 95, no. 5 (May 2019): 1053–1063

Al-Balas, Alian, Timmy Lee, Carlton J. Young, Jill Barker-Finkel, and Michael Allon. "Predictors of Initiation for Predialysis Arteriovenous Fistula." *Clinical Journal of the American Society of Nephrology* 11, no. 10 (October 7, 2016): 1802–8. https://doi.org/10.2215/cjn.00700116.

Allon, Michael. "Vascular Access for Hemodialysis Patients: New Data Should Guide Decision Making." *Clinical Journal of the American Society of Nephrology* 14, no. 6 (June 7, 2019): 954–61. https://doi.org/10.2215/cjn.00490119.

Dixon, Bradley S. "Timing of Arteriovenous Fistula Placement: Keeping It in Perspective." *Journal of the American Society of Nephrology* 26, no. 2 (February 2015): 241–43. https://doi.org/10.1681/asn.2014070709.

Ferrari, Paolo. "Nurturing the Benefits of Pre-Emptive Kidney Transplantation." *Nephrology Dialysis Transplantation* 31, no. 5 (November 14, 2015): 681–82. https://doi.org/10.1093/ndt/gfv383.

Grams, Morgan E., Allan B. Massie, Josef Coresh, and Dorry L. Segev. "Trends in the Timing of Pre-emptive Kidney Transplantation." *Journal of the American Society of Nephrology* 22, no. 9 (September 2011): 1615–20. https://doi.

org/10.1681/asn.2011010023.

Helmick, Ryan A., Colleen L. Jay, Brittany A. Price, Patrick G. Dean, and Mark D. Stegall. "Identifying Barriers to Preemptive Kidney Transplantation in a Living Donor Transplant Cohort." *Transplantation Direct* 4, no. 4 (March 19, 2018): e356. https://doi.org/10.1097/txd.0000000000000773.

Jay, Colleen L., Patrick G. Dean, Ryan A. Helmick, and Mark D. Stegall. "Reassessing Preemptive Kidney Transplantation in the United States." *Transplantation* 100, no. 5 (May 2016): 1120–27. https://doi.org/10.1097/tp.0000000000000944.

Molnar, Miklos Z., Akinlolu O. Ojo, Suphamai Bunnapradist, Csaba P. Kovesdy, and Kamyar Kalantar-Zadeh. "Timing of Dialysis Initiation in Transplant-Naive and Failed Transplant Patients." *Nature Reviews Nephrology* 8, no. 5 (February 28, 2012): 284–92. https://doi.org/10.1038/nrneph.2012.36.

Santoro, Domenico, Filippo Benedetto, Placido Mondello, Francesco Spinelli, Carlo Alberto Ricciardi, Valeria Cernaro, Michele Buemi, Narayana Pipitò, and David Barillà. "Vascular Access for Hemodialysis: Current Perspectives." *International Journal of Nephrology and Renovascular Disease* 7 (July 8, 2014): 281–94. https://doi.org/10.2147/ijnrd.s46643.

Sukul, Nidhi, Junhui Zhao, Douglas S. Fuller, Angelo Karaboyas, Brian Bieber, James A. Sloand, Lalita Subramanian, et al. "Patient-

Reported Advantages and Disadvantages of Peritoneal Dialysis: Results from the PDOPPS." *BMC Nephrology* 20, no. 1 (April 2, 2019): 116. https://doi.org/10.1186/s12882-019-1304-3.

Wiseman, Alexander C. "Protecting Donors and Safeguarding Altruism in the United States." *Clinical Journal of the American Society of Nephrology* 13, no. 5 (March 2018): 790–92. https://doi.org/10.2215/cjn.13681217.

Woo, Karen, Dana P. Goldman, and John A. Romley. "Early Failure of Dialysis Access among the Elderly in the Era of Fistula First." *Clinical Journal of the American Society of Nephrology* 10, no. 10 (October 7, 2015): 1791–98. https://doi.org/10.2215/cjn.09040914.

Zhou, Hui, John J. Sim, Simran K. Bhandari, Sally F. Shaw, Jiaxiao Shi, Scott A. Rasgon, Csaba P. Kovesdy, Kamyar Kalantar-Zadeh, Michael H. Kanter, and Steven J. Jacobsen. "Early Mortality Among Peritoneal Dialysis and Hemodialysis Patients Who Transitioned With an Optimal Outpatient Start." *Kidney International Reports* 4, no. 2 (October 16, 2018): 275–84. https://doi.org/10.1016/j.ekir.2018.10.008.

# Index

**Page ranges in bold refer to Dr. Ro's Pearls of Wisdom.**

A1C levels, 35, 79

access points

    for hemodialysis, 139, 152, 154, 155, 156–159

    for peritoneal dialysis, 149, 150, 151

ACE (angiotensin-converting enzyme) inhibitors

    for glomerular disease, 69

    for high blood pressure, 72

    precautions when using, 81, 101, 106

    for proteinuria, 69, 72, 73–74

    temporary eGFR drops caused by, 58–60, 62–63, 74–75

acetaminophen (Tylenol), 81, 82

acidosis, 96–98, 120–121

activated vitamin D (calcitriol), 117, 119, 120

acute kidney injury (AKI). *See reversible kidney function declines*

acute tubular necrosis (ATN), 55, 56–58

Adderall, 72

adult-onset diabetes (type 2), 66. See also diabetes

advanced chronic kidney disease

    anemias and, 111–115, 121–122, **176–177**. *See also anemias*

    defined, 85

    electrolyte management for, 95–110, **174–176**. See also electrolyte management

    mineral and bone diseases related to, 115–122, **177–178**. *See also* chronic kidney disease mineral and bone disorder

NSAIDs precautions for, 81–82

renal replacement therapy options, 123. *See also* dialysis; kidney transplant

Smart Diet modifications for, 51–52

Advil (ibuprofen), 58, 81–82. *See also* NSAIDs

African Americans, 68

age, rate of kidney function decline and, 88–89. *See also* older adults

AKI (acute kidney injury). *See* reversible kidney function declines

albumin, 17, 97

albuminuria, 17, 20, 21

Aldactone (spironolactone), 100. *See* also potassium-sparing diuretics

Aleve, 58. *See* also NSAIDs

Aleve (naproxen), 82. See also NSAIDs

alkali therapy, 79–80

alkalosis, 96

amiloride (Midamor), 100. *See also* potassium-sparing diuretics

anemias, 111–115

    about, 111

    causes, 112–113

    diagnosing, 113

    summary, 121–122, **176–177**

    symptoms, 114

    treatment, 114–115

angiotensin-converting enzyme inhibitors. *See* ACE inhibitors

antacids, 60, 114, 117. *See also* calcium-containing phosphorus binders

A1C levels, 35, 79

ARBs (angiotensin-receptor blockers)

for glomerular disease, 69

for high blood pressure, 72

precautions when using, 81, 101, 106

for proteinuria, 69, 72, 73–74

reversible kidney function declines caused by, 58–60, 62–63, 74–75

aristolochic acid, 3, 53

arterial calcification, 116, 117

aspirin, 81, 82, 83

atherosclerosis, 25–37

about, 25–26

as cause of kidney disease, 68

lifestyle changes for avoiding, 2–3, 26–36, 40, 46–47

management of, 73–74

metabolic acidosis and, 97

risk factors, 2–3, 20–21, 27–34, 36, 46–47, 66

Smart Diet and, 2, 40, 46

summary, 37, **166–167**

symptoms, 26

ATN (acute tubular necrosis), 55, 56–58

atorvastatin (Lipitor), 34

AV (arteriovenous) access, 139, 152, 154, 155, 156–159

AV (arteriovenous) fistula, 139, 154, 156–158, 159

azilsartan, 59, 101. *See also* ARBs


baby aspirin, 83

Bactrim (sulfamethoxazole and trimethoprim), 101

"bad" cholesterol (LDL), 29, 33–34, 45, 46

baking soda (sodium bicarbonate), 3, 79–80, 97–98, 101, 121

benazepril, 59, 101. See also ACE inhibitors

benign prostatic hypertrophy, 63

beverages

    alcoholic, 44, 72

    caffeinated, 44

    sugary, 43, 51

bicarbonate levels, 95–96, 97–98, 120

bladder, 11, 63–64

bleeding, CKD-related, 136

blood, in urine, 16, 17–20

blood creatinine. *See* serum creatinine

blood pH, 12, 96, 98

blood pressure. *See also* high blood pressure; low blood pressure

    protocol for accurate readings, 31

    target blood pressures, 31–32, 70–71

blood pressure medications, 30–32, 57, 58–60, 71–72. *See also* ACE inhibitors; ARBs

blood sugar control, 35–36, 45, 66–67, 78–79, 97

blood transfusions, 112, 115, 147

bone disorders. *See* chronic kidney disease mineral and bone disorder

Buchwald, Art, 57

bumetanide (Bumex), 107. *See also* loop diuretics

caffeinated beverages, 44

calcified blood vessels, 116, 117

calcimimetics, 119

calcitriol (Rocaltrol or activated vitamin D), 117, 119, 120

calcium-containing phosphorus binders (antacids), 60, 114, 117, 119

calcium levels, 12, 95–96, 115–116, 119, 120

calorie intake, 34, 40, 41–45

canagliflozin, 67

candesartan, 59, 101. *See also* ARBs

canned foods, 51, 102

CAPD (continuous ambulatory peritoneal dialysis), 149

captopril, 59. *See also* ACE inhibitors

carbohydrate intake, 41, 43–46

carbon dioxide, 96, 97

causes, of CKD, 66–72

    atherosclerosis, 68. *See also* atherosclerosis

    diabetic kidney disease, 66–67. *See also* diabetes

    glomerular diseases, 68–69

    hypertensive nephropathy, 67–68. *See also* high blood pressure

    polycystic kidney disease, 69–70

CBC (complete blood count), 113

Celebrex, 58. *See also* NSAIDs

central venous catheter (CVC access), 154, 158, 159

CHF. *See* congestive heart failure

Chinese herbs, 3

chloride levels, 95, 98

chlorthalidone (Diuril), 107. *See also* thiazide diuretics

cholesterol levels, 29, 33–34, 45, 46

chronic kidney disease (CKD)

    associated disorders, 111–122. See also anemias; atherosclerosis; chronic kidney disease mineral and bone disorder; diabetes

    causes of, 66–72.*See also* causes, of CKD

    diagnosis, 13, 23. *See also* estimated glomerular filtration rate; glomerular filtration rate

    management of, 65–84, 139–161. *See also* dialysis; kidney

transplant; management, of CKD

myths about, 19

overdiagnosis of, 19

prevalence, 1

prognosis, 3–4. *See also* kidney function declines

stages of, 18–23. *See also* stages, of chronic kidney disease

symptoms, lack of, 4, 19

chronic kidney disease mineral and bone disorder (CKD-MBD), 115–121

about, 115–116

fracture rates and, 120

metabolic acidosis and, 120–121

protein intake and, 47–48

summary, 121–122, **177–178**

treatment recommendations, 117–120

cinacalcet hydrochloride (Sensipar), 119. See also vitamin D drugs

CKD. See chronic kidney disease

CKD-MBD. See chronic kidney disease mineral and bone disorder

Clark, W., 80

complete blood count (CBC), 113

congestive heart failure (CHF)

anemia and, 114

early start of dialysis due to, 132, 135

hemodialysis and, 153

management of, 106

patient example, 109

precautions for, 79–80, 81, 97–98, 100

reversible kidney function declines and, 62–63

continuous ambulatory peritoneal dialysis (CAPD), 149
creatinine. *See* serum creatinine; urine
creatinine clearance, 14–15, 80, 130–131
CVC access (central venous catheter), 154, 158, 159

dapagliflozin, 67
dehydration, 56–57, 58, 61, 80–81
diabetes
    atherosclerosis risk and, 36, 66
    bladder-emptying problems, 64
    blood sugar control for, 3, 35–36, 79
    cholesterol level goals for, 33–34, 46
    diabetic kidney disease (nephropathy), 66–67, 68, 79
    diabetic retinopathy, 35, 36, 66–67
    dialysis guidelines for, 134
    diet recommendations, 39, 44, 45, 75–76
    eye exams for, 36
    foot care for, 36
    glomerular disease and, 69
    hyperkalemia and, 99
    prevention, 34, 44, 45
    type 1 and type 2, 66
diabetic kidney disease (nephropathy), 66–67, 68, 79
diabetic retinopathy, 35, 36, 66–67
dialysis
    about, 87, 125–126, 139–140
    for acute kidney injury, 55, 57–58, 90–91, 131–132, 135
    AV access and, 139, 152, 154, 155, 156–159
    delaying dialysis, patient examples, 93–94, 109, 127–128

delaying dialysis, with electrolyte management, 95–110, **174–176**. *See also* electrolyte management

dialysis-free years calculation, 90

early start trend history, 126–129, 132–133

kidney failure risk equation (KFRE), 91–92

kidney transplant option versus, 123, 139–140, 141

kidney transplant timing and, 145–147

options for, 148–159. *See also* hemodialysis; home dialysis; peritoneal dialysis

potential harm from, 88–89, 92–94, 128–130, 141

predicting factors, 62–63, 66, 68, 70, 90–94, 99, 106, 173–174

recovery of kidney function during, 57–58, 90–91

side effects, 129–130

stages of CKD and, 18, 21, 23

start guidelines, 4–5, 15, 19–21, 56, 94, 130–136

statistics on, 1, 66, 68, 69, 70

summary, 94, 136–137, 160–161, 173–176, 178–180, 182–184

survival advantage with, 92–94, 128

diclofenac (Voltaren), 82

diuretics

about, 107

for congestive heart failure, 62–63, 132

delaying dialysis and, 107–109

for high blood pressure, 72, 73–74

for hyperkalemia, 101

patient example, 109

precautions when using, 56, 62–63, 98, 100, 107, 132

summary, 109–110

Diuril (chlorthalidone), 107. *See also* thiazide diuretics

doxercalciferol (Hectorol), 119. *See also* vitamin D drugs

Dyrenium (triamterene), 100. *See also* potassium-sparing
  diuretics

e-cigarettes, 28

Edecrin (ethacrynic acid), 107. See also loop diuretics

eGFR. See estimated glomerular filtration rate

electrolyte management, 95–110

  about, 95–96

  alkalosis, 96

  diuretics and, 107–109

  electrolyte, defined, 95

  electrolyte report, defined, 95

  hyperkalemia, 98, 99–106, 135. See also hyperkalemia

  hypokalemia, 106–107

  metabolic acidosis, 96–98, 120–131

  metabolic alkalosis, 98

  patient example, 109

  summary, 109–110, **174–176**

empagliflozin, 67

enalapril, 59, 101. *See also* ACE inhibitors

end-stage renal disease, 19–21. *See also* dialysis; kidney transplant; stages, of chronic kidney disease

eplerenone (Inspra), 100. *See also* potassium-sparing diuretics

eprosartan, 59, 101. See also ARBs

erythropoietin (EPO), 112, 115

esomeprazole (Nexium), 60

estimated glomerular filtration rate (eGFR)

  about, 7, 12–13

  accuracy of, 15, 19, 130–131

ACE inhibitors' and ARBs' effect on, 69, 74–75, 106

atherosclerosis and, 68

blood sugar levels and, 35

calculation of, 14–15

CKD-related bone disease and, 116, 118, 120

dialysis guidelines based on, 132–135, 136

diuretics' effect on, 108–109

erythropoietin and, 113

hemodialysis access timing based on, 159

hypertension and, 67, 71

kidney transplant guidelines based on, 143, 147

normal ranges, 13

normal rate of loss, 89

NSAIDs' effect on, 81–82

in older adults, 88–89

reversible drops in. See reversible kidney function declines

stages of CKD based on, 18–23

summary, 23–24, **163–165**

ethacrynic acid (Edecrin), 107. See also loop diuretics

exercising, 32, 42, 44–45, 120

eye exams, 36

fats (dietary), 41, 46

Feldene (piroxicam), 82

fenofibrate (TriCor), 34

ferrous fumarate, 114–115

ferrous gluconate, 114–115

ferrous sulfate, 114–115

fiber, 44, 45–46

fibric acid drugs, 34
folic acid deficiency, 112, 115
food labels, 41–44, 45–46, 47, 49
FoodSwitch app, 118
foot care, 36
fosinopril, 59, 101. See also ACE inhibitors
fractures, 77, 116, 120
furosemide (Lasix), 107. See also loop diuretics

gamipril, 59
gastroesophageal reflux (GERD), 60–61
gemfibrozil, 34
"-gliflozin" drugs, 67
glomerular disease, 68–69
glomerular filtrate, 10
glomerular filtration rate (measured), 14–16, 23, 130–131
glomerulus, 10, 16, 17
"good" cholesterol (HDL), 33–34
graft, for AV access, 158

hardening of arteries. See atherosclerosis
HDL ("good" cholesterol), 33–34
heart attacks
    A1C target levels and, 35
    aspirin for prevention of, 83
    hemoglobin levels and, 115
    smoking and, 27
    symptoms, 26
heart failure. See congestive heart failure
Hectorol (doxercalciferol), 119. See also vitamin D drugs

hemodialysis, 151–159
    access issues, 139, 152, 154, 155, 156–159
    in-center, 152–154
    diet recommendations, 151–152
    at home, 148, 155
    incremental hemodialysis, 154–155
hemoglobin, 111, 112, 113, 115
hemoglobin A1C test, 35, 79
heparin, 101
herbal supplements, 3, 53–54
high blood pressure (hypertension)
    atherosclerosis risk factor, 25
    diagnosis, 23
    erythropoietin injections and, 115
    kidney disease and, 67–68, 70–72, 74–75
    management of, 30–31, 47, 59, 70–72. See also ACE inhibitors; ARBs
    metabolic acidosis and, 97
    patient example, 74–75
    target blood pressures, 31–32, 70–71
    "white coat" hypertension, 30, 72
Hispanic Americans, 70
home dialysis
    hemodialysis, 148, 152
    as kidney transplant alternative, 139
    peritoneal dialysis, 148–151, 153–154, 160
hydration, 56–57, 58, 61, 80–81
hydrochlorothiazide (HCTZ or HydroDiuril), 101, 107
hyperkalemia

about, 99–100
causes, 100–101, 106
diet recommendations, 102–105
early start of dialysis due to, 135
metabolic alkalosis treatment and, 98
resistant hyperkalemia, 105–106, 135
symptoms, 99
hypertension. See high blood pressure
hypertensive nephropathy, 67–68
hypoglycemia, 79
hypokalemia, 106–107
hypotension. See low blood pressure

ibuprofen (Motrin or Advil), 58, 81–82. See also NSAIDs
idiopathic glomerular diseases, 69
indapamide (Lozol), 107. See also thiazide diuretics
indomethacin (Indocin), 82. See also NSAIDs
inherited kidney diseases, 68, 69–70
Inspra (eplerenone), 100. See also potassium-sparing diuretics
intravenous x-ray contrast tests, 61
irbesartan, 59, 101. See also ARBs
iron-deficiency anemia, 112–115
iron supplementation, 114–115

Kayexalate (sodium polystyrene), 105–106
ketoanalogues, 78
ketoprofen (Orudis), 82. See also NSAIDs
KFRE (kidney failure risk equation), 91–92
kidney anatomy, 9–11

kidney failure. See end-stage renal disease
kidney failure risk equation (KFRE), 91–92
kidney function declines
    diet recommendations, 2
    lifestyle changes for avoiding, 2–3
    measure of, 7, 12–13, 16. See also estimated glomerular
      filtration rate; glomerular filtration rate
    predictors of, 71, 73–74, 91–94
    progression of, 4–5
    reversible, 8, 55–64. See also reversible kidney function
      declines
    speed of, 70–72. See also speed of kidney function decline
kidney stones, 63–64, 81
kidney transplant, 139–161
    about, 123, 139–140
    cadaver donor transplant, 147–148
    dialysis versus, 123, 139–140, 141
    eligibility for, 140–141, 143–148
    live donor transplant, 143–147
    long term risks, 142–143
    preemptive transplant issues, 145–147
    pretransplant workup, 143
    rejection of, 142
    summary, 160–161, **180–182**
    surgical procedure details, 142

labels (food), 41–44
labetalol, 101
lansoprazole (Prevacid), 60
Lasix (furosemide), 107. See also loop diuretics

LDL ("bad" cholesterol), 29, 33–34, 45, 46

leaching, of vegetables, 102–103

Lipitor (atorvastatin), 34

lisinopril, 59, 101. See also ACE inhibitors

"Lite Salt," 47, 100, 102

Lokelma (sodium zirconium), 106

loop diuretics, 101, 107–108

losartan, 59, 101. See also ARBs

low blood pressure (hypotension)

    with in-center hemodialysis, 153–154

    kidney function declines and, 32, 57, 71

    target blood pressures, 31–32, 70–71

low blood sugar levels, 35–36, 79

low-carb diet, 43–44

low-fat diet, 46

low-phosphorus diet, 118

low-potassium diets, 102–105

low-protein diet

    about, 1–3, 48, 75–78

    malnutrition issues, 47–48

    overemphasis on, 39

    Smart Diet versus, 49

    very-low-protein diet, 1–3, 8, 40, 47–49, 65, 75–78

Lozol (indapamide), 107. See also thiazide diuretics


macroalbuminuria, 17, 74

management, of CKD, 65–84

    blood pressure control and, 30–31, 47, 59, 70–72. See also
      ACE inhibitors; ARBs

blood sugar control and, 35–36, 45, 66–67, 78–79, 97

diet recommendations, 39–41. *See also* low-protein diet; Smart Diet

electrolyte management, 95–110. *See also* electrolyte management

exercising, 32, 42, 44–45, 120

glomerular disease and, 69

multidisciplinary follow-up, 36, 65–66

overview, 65

polycystic kidney disease and, 69–70

renal replacement therapy options. *See* dialysis; kidney transplant

summary, 83–84, 171–173

urine protein levels and, 73–74

measured glomerular filtration rate, 14–16, 23, 130–131

Medicare coverage, 126, 141, 145

meditation, 32

metabolic acidosis, 96–98, 120–121

metabolic alkalosis, 98

metolazone (Zaroxolyn), 107

microalbuminuria, 17

Midamor (amiloride), 100.*See also* potassium-sparing diuretics

mineral disorders. See chronic kidney disease mineral and bone disorder

moexipril, 59, 101. See also ACE inhibitors

Motrin (ibuprofen), 58, 81–82. See also NSAIDs

muscle loss (wasting), 52, 77, 97

muscle-strengthening exercises, 29, 45, 120

naproxen (Aleve), 82. See also NSAIDs

nephron, 9–10
Nexium (esomeprazole), 60
NKF Peers Lending Support Program, 147
NSAIDs (nonsteroidal anti-inflammatory drugs), 58, 60, 81–82, 101
Nurofen, 82

obesity, 2, 25, 34, 40, 141
older adults
    kidney function decline rate of, 88–89
    muscle loss and, 52, 77
    Smart Diet modifications, 52
    social isolation and, 32
omeprazole (Prilosec), 60
opiates, 82
Orudis (ketoprofen), 82.See also NSAIDs
osteoporosis, 97, 120, 121
"over diuresis," 62

paired donor exchange program, 144–145
parathyroidectomy, 120
parathyroid hormone (PTH), 116, 119–120
paricalcitol (Zemplar), 119.See also vitamin D drugs
patiromer (Veltassa), 105–106
PCKD (polycystic kidney disease), 69–70
pericarditis, 136
perindopril, 59
peritoneal dialysis (PD), 148–151, 153–154, 160
Phoslo (antacid), 114, 117. See also calcium-containing phosphorus binders

phosphorus binders, 12, 95–96, 115–116, 118–119, 120
phosphorus levels, 12, 47, 49, 51–52, 116–120
piroxicam (Feldene), 82
plasma, 11
polycystic kidney disease (PCKD), 69–70
polyunsaturated fats, 46
potassium-binding medication, 105–106
potassium chloride, 47
potassium chloride tablets, 98, 107
potassium levels
    CBC and, 95
    elevated levels, 98, 99–105, 106, 135
    low levels, 106–107
    low-potassium diets, 47, 102–105
    metabolic acidosis and, 97
    metabolic alkalosis and, 98
    resistant hyperkalemia, 105–106, 135
    summary, 109–110, **174–176**
potassium-sparing diuretics, 100, 107
PPIs (proton pump inhibitors), 60–61
Prevacid (lansoprazole), 60
"-pril" drugs. *See* ACE inhibitors
Prilosec (omeprazole), 60
processed foods, 51, 102, 118–119
propranolol, 101
prostate enlargement, 63
protein intake. *See* low-protein diet; Smart Diet; very-low-protein diet
proteinuria (protein in urine)
    atherosclerosis and, 27, 36

glomerular disease and, 68–69

management of, 35, 73–74, 77–78

measurement of, 15, 16–17

as predictor of kidney function loss, 71, 73–74, 91–94

staging of CKD based on, 20–22

target blood pressures for, 71

proton pump inhibitors (PPIs), 60–61

PTH (parathyroid hormone), 116, 119–120


quinapril, 59, 101. *See also* ACE inhibitors


race, 68, 70

rapid kidney function decline. *See* reversible kidney function
  declines; speed of kidney function decline

recipe resources, 52

red blood cell transfusion, 112, 115

rejection, of kidney transplant, 142

renal pelvis, 11

renal replacement therapy. See dialysis; kidney transplant

resistant hyperkalemia, 105–106, 135

respiratory acidosis, 96

respiratory alkalosis, 96

reversible kidney function declines (acute kidney failure), 55–64

  about, 55

  acute tubular necrosis, 55, 56–58

  causes, 55–64

  defined, 8

  dehydration and, 56–57, 58, 61

  dialysis for, 55, 57–58, 90–91, 131–132, 135

  low blood pressure and, 32, 57

medications as cause of, 58–63, 74–75

prostate enlargement and, 63

repeat eGFRs for, 55, 58–60, 62–64

summary, 64, **170–171**

urine flow blockage and, 63–64

Ritalin, 72

Rocaltrol (calcitriol or activated vitamin D), 117, 119, 120

Rolaids (antacid), 60, 114

salt intake, 47, 72

saturated fats, 46

seizures, 136

Sensipar (cinacalcet hydrochloride), 119. See also vitamin D drugs

serum creatinine. See also creatinine clearance; urine: creatinine levels

about, 7, 12–13

creatinine clearance calculation based on, 14–15

diuretics' effect on, 108–109

eGFR calculation based on, 12–13, 18–19, 130–131

home remedy precautions, 14

SGLT2 inhibitors, 67

short-acting NSAIDs, 81–82

simvastatin (Zocor), 34

skin cancer, 142

sleep apnea, 33

Smart Diet

about, 2, 8, 39–41, 76

advanced CKD modifications, 51–52

beverage recommendations, 43–44

on carbohydrate intake, 41, 43–46

for CKD-MBD, 120–121

on diet supplements, 53–54

for electrolyte management, 49, 80, 97–98, 105, 118–119, 120–121

on fat intake, 41, 46

on fiber intake, 44, 45–46

on food labels, 41–44

for older adults, 52

on protein intake, 41, 44, 47–49, 50

recipe resources, 52

recommended foods, 50–51

on salt intake, 47

on sugar intake, 43, 46

summary, 54, 167–169

total daily calories, 41–43

smoking cessation, 27–28

social isolation, 32

sodium bicarbonate pills, 79–80, 97–98, 101, 121

sodium chloride/saline IV, 98

sodium intake, 47, 72

sodium polystyrene (Kayexalate), 105–106

sodium zirconium (Lokelma), 106

speed of kidney function decline

alkali therapy, 3, 79–80

blood pressure control and, 70–72

blood sugar control and, 78–79

dietary considerations, 75–78

management of, 75–81

protein in urine and, 71, 73–74, 91–94

race and, 70

summary, 83–84, 171–173

water consumption, 80–81

spironolactone (Aldactone), 100. *See also* potassium-sparing
  diuretics

spot urine tests, 16–17, 21, 73, 77

stages, of chronic kidney disease, 18–23

current classification, 20–22

defined, 18

glomerular filtration rate pattern change versus, 23

misinformation on, 19

problems with, 18–20

prognosis based on, 4, 23

rationale for, 2–3

statistics, 22

treatment recommendations based on, 22

statins, 33–34

stress relief, 32

stroke, 26, 35, 83

sugar intake, 43, 46

sulfamethoxazole and trimethoprim (Bactrim), 101

supplements

guidelines, 3, 8, 53–54

for iron deficiency, 114–115

keto-acid supplements, 78


"-tan" drugs. *See* ARBs

telmisartan, 59, 101. *See also* ARBs

thiazide diuretics, 101, 107–108

Timing of Clinical Outcomes in CKD with Severely Decreased GFR, 92

tolvaptan, 70. *See also* ARBs

topical NSAIDs, 82

trandolapril, 59, 101. *See also* ACE inhibitors

transferrin saturation scores, 113

triamterene (Dyrenium), 100. See also potassium-sparing diuretics

TriCor (fenofibrate), 34

Tums (antacid), 60, 114, 117. See also calcium-containing phosphorus binders

Tylenol (acetaminophen), 81, 82

type 1 and type 2 diabetes, 66. *See also* diabetes


ureters, 11

urethra, 11

urine

    albumin levels, 17, 20, 21

    blockage of, 63–64

    blood in, 16, 17–20

    collection, 15, 16, 17, 73

    creatinine levels, 14–15, 17, 80, 130–131

    formation, 10–11

    protein levels, 15, 16–17, 20–22. *See also* proteinuria

urine dipstick, 16–17


valsartan, 59, 101. *See also* ARBs

vaping, 28

vein mapping, 157

vein preservation, 157

Veltassa (patiromer), 105–106

very-low-protein diet, 1–3, 8, 40, 47–49, 65, 75–78
vision loss, 35, 36, 67
vitamin B12 deficiency, 112, 115
vitamin D deficiency, 116, 117
vitamin D drugs, 117, 119, 120
Voltaren (diclofenac), 82

water intake, 44, 56–57, 58, 61, 80–81
water pills. *See* diuretics
weight loss, 32, 34, 40–45, 120
"white coat" hypertension, 30, 72

x-ray contrast tests, 61

Zaroxolyn (metolazone), 107
Zemplar (paricalcitol), 119. See also vitamin D drugs
Zocor (simvastatin), 34

Made in United States
Troutdale, OR
10/17/2023